FUEL YOUR BODY NATURALLY

BE A LONG-LASTING ENDURANCE MACHINE

DR. SAMTA MAHAJAN & SUNIL MENON

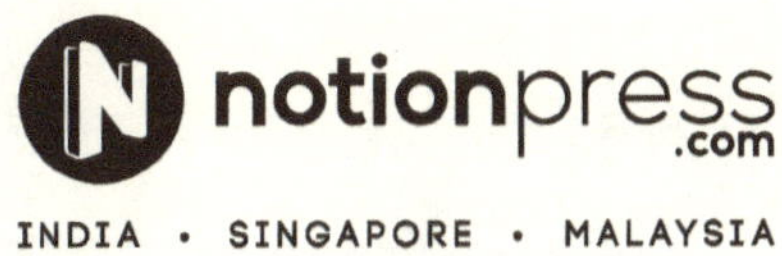

Notion Press

No. 8, 3rd Cross Street,
CIT Colony, Mylapore,
Chennai, Tamil Nadu – 600 004

First Published by Notion Press 2021
Copyright © Menon Fitness 2021
All Rights Reserved.

ISBN 978-1-63806-787-0

Dedication

To every champion who reads this book.

Disclaimer

The information presented in this book is not intended to replace an Ayurvedic practitioner or nutritionist/dietician in case of a disease. If you have any medical condition, do consult your doctor. As the treatment and diet plan is unique for each person with their specific constitution, it requires close supervision.

Contents

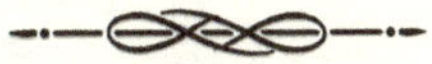

Evolution of Food Habits

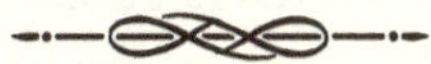

"As humans, we have progressed through multiple revolutions, but we have forgotten how natural food tastes. I hope to see a green revolution where humans and nature co-exist, and the future generations enjoy the unadulterated taste of food."

Hippocrates' philosophy to use "Food as Medicine" is a growing interest in the science of food. When human species appeared on Earth, environmental conditions must have been favorable for its survival. Many years ago, the man survived by hunting animals, picking wild fruits, vegetables, roots, and shoots. Over the past few decades, there have been several dietary changes in human evolution. Over the period, there was a shift from hunter-gatherer times to agricultural times to industrial civilization. Due to these changes, our eating habits have substantially changed. It makes us wonder how they were able to get all the nutritious food needed for an active person at that time. Today, most of us are thinking of getting energy from sugar, protein powders, and supplements. Let's have a brief look at how our Stone Age ancestors evolved from hunter-gatherers to industrial civilization.

Paleolithic period (2.5 million years ago)- This period is also called the **Old Stone Age,** as the human species made tools and weapons out of stone. There were only two ways of obtaining food, either by hunting or by gathering. During this period, the food available was meat, wild plants, vegetables, fungi, roots, shoots, fruits, and nuts. In the lower paleolithic period, they included fishing and hunting. Their diet varied according to the season and availability of foods. The ratio of the fat content that they consumed differed from what we consume today. The Omega-6 to Omega-3 ratio was about 3:1 compared to 12:1 what we take. Free-range animals have about five times more polyunsaturated fat compared to supermarket meat. The overall nutritional quality of food the stone age people ate was appropriate to their kind. Paleolithic humans were taller, had strongly built bodies with erect posture. The paleolithic diet did not contain grains, dairy, lentils, or legumes.[1]

Fire has been in use as early as about 1.5 million years ago, but these fires could have been wildfires instead of human-made fire. The control of fire by early humans was a turning point in the cultural aspect of evolution. Fire helped them stay warm, cook meats and vegetables, and keep predators away. Before the discovery of control fire, man was confined to warmer climates. After invention, he may have been able to migrate to colder places. Fire increased the average life span. Cooking allowed to eat more palatable meals and also allowed to kill unhealthy bacteria present in raw meat.

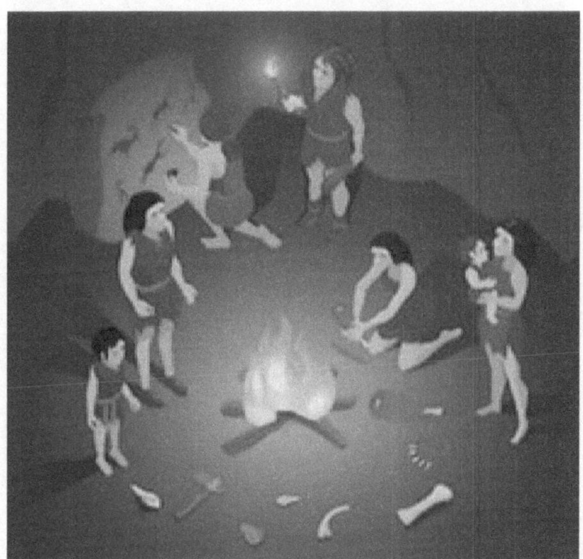

Picture 1: Primitive ancient people

Neolithic period (10,000 years ago) – Neolithic period was also called New Stone Age, as humans were still using stone tools, but they were more refined and polished. As the climate changed from Ice Age to much warmer conditions, vegetation flourished. This period was marked by a transition from hunting and gathering to farming. People were no longer food gatherers, but they became food producers. Hence, this period is also called the agriculture revolution. Due to farming, they started settling in one place. Cereal cultivation and animal domestication were introduced. They started to store food.

Food available was wheat, barley, rice, maize, legumes, lentils, vegetables, fruits, wild plants, nuts, and roots. This was a shift to the grain-based diet from the paleolithic era.

Neolithic diet always encourages people to eat a basic and healthy diet. There was no processed food at that time, but their nutrition was inferior compared to hunters' gatherers. Dental cavities became known for the first time during the Neolithic period as there were nutritional deficiencies. The health of people of the Neolithic era was much better compared to today's generation. [2]

Industrial Revolution

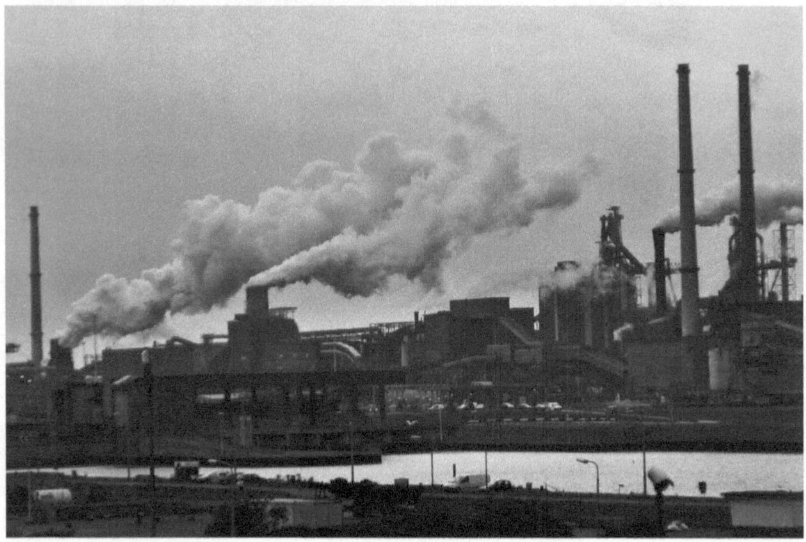

Picture 2: Industrial revolution

The population increased due to better sanitation and medicine, which led to longer life spans. This resulted in a high rate of population growth, so they started looking for more work. Many industries, factories emerged during this period, and the prehistoric lifestyle got changed completely. During the middle ages, the whole day was structured quite differently than it is today. People got up much earlier and went to bed much earlier. During that time, as there was no electricity, people ate only during the daytime. After the invention of electricity, dinner shifted much later in the day.

A few decades ago, people used to eat two meals a day. When people transited from farms to factories, they had to leave early from their houses, resulting in the breakfast culture. Breakfast allowed them to sustain for long working hours in harsh conditions. Moreover, when breakfast cereal got invented, they emphasized eating cereal. [3]

It started with the plain old cereals, but adding sugars, other additives, and preservatives ended up making it a highly processed food item. Breakfast means you are breaking the fast as you are eating after 6-8 hours. As our digestive fire stays low in the morning, light foods are recommended. So, the first meal of the day should be light and healthy. Fruits, nuts, sprouts, porridge, or warm-cooked light meals are consumed. Consuming fruits at the beginning of the day is the best way to get maximum nutritional benefits.

Processed and GMO food – With the invention of machinery, there was more production of refined flour, refined vegetable oils, and ready-to-eat snacks, which are highly deteriorating for health. The shift from whole grains to refined flour directly impacted nutrient intake, as refined flour deprives of many nutrients. With the industrial revolution, people started eating more sugar and trans fats. They reduced their fiber content, which is a massive change from our prehistoric ancestors' diet. Family farms were replaced with large fields of genetically modified crops, which started the usage of pesticides. Genetically modified organisms are food crops whose genetic makeup has been altered using genetic engineering. This increases the allergens and other toxins. After using genetically modified food, people start getting allergies, joint pains, gluten sensitivities, anxiety, depression, etc.

In agricultural areas, families were bound to eat only what they could grow. As agriculture brought in less income to the household, families preferred to shift to industries to earn a good income. Due to a shortage of agricultural land, unpredictable weather conditions, and more income from industries, many families moved to urban areas. The industrial revolution regularized working hours. Some had to leave early for work, so the canteen concept came into the limelight during this period. As the workers worked further away from their homes, they could not go home for a mid-day meal. In that case, the solution was to buy lunch from outside. Food which otherwise would be eaten fresh started being conserved so that it can be used shortly. Instead of consuming fresh produce, people started preserving it by adding excess salt and other preservatives.

Urbanization also brought in the concept of eating food outside the house under budgetary constraints. The fast-food industry evolved to give access to lesser-priced food. Exposure to a modern diet and a sedentary lifestyle resulted in an increased risk of developing obesity, diabetes, and coronary heart diseases. Elevated homocysteine levels in the blood are linked to an increased risk of Coronary heart disease and stroke. Homocysteine levels rise when Vitamin B and folic acid are insufficient, and refined flour is deficient in these nutrients. The typical modern diet contains more starch, sugar, and less fiber than the prehistoric human diet. High sodium and low potassium diet are typically seen in modern diets. [4] food processing techniques have changed in this generation. These changing dietary patterns are mainly responsible for the decline of human health, and it is only getting worse.

Moreover, we are bombarded with advertisements that show where to get the best pizzas, burgers, fries, and candies. Children are fascinated by colorful advertisements of packaged foods with their favorite cartoon characters printed on them, which has an intrinsic value to attract attention. The purpose of advertisements is to try to make you buy something. Don't be an impulsive buyer. Always think before buying. Watch this as entertainment and do not take it seriously. They are just marketing gimmicks.

From the prehistoric era till now, we have changed our eating habits significantly. From fresh produce to canned and packaged products, we have shifted from jaggery to sugar, from cold-pressed oils to refined oils, from fresh juices to bottled juices. These changes that we have adapted to are only taking us into a health disaster.

However, nowadays, the produce is not the same as our ancestors ate but still, we have access to organic vegetables and fruits.

It's better to shift our food habits back to what our ancestors had. Back to roots will only make us healthy.

Gut (Our Second Brain)

"I hope we tune-in to our Gut feeling and make the right choice of food habits. Let's enrich the biodiversity of our gut; let's make it colorful."

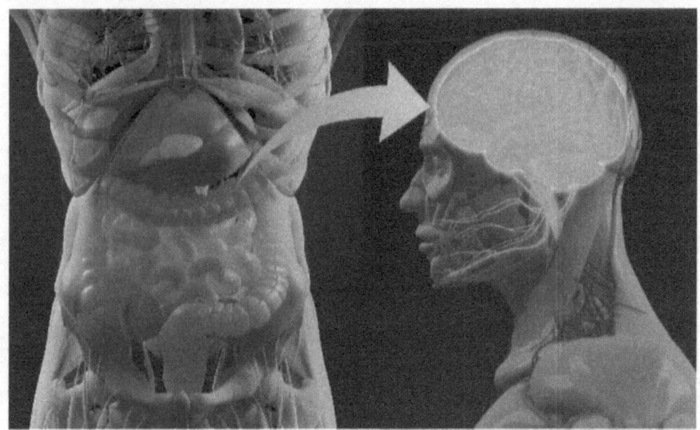

Picture 3: Gut to brain signal and vice versa

We experience butterflies in our stomachs when we are nervous. Our elders always said listen to your gut feeling. These are signals from our second brain. This second brain is hidden in our digestive system, which we call the "Gut." Gut talks to the brain and vice versa. Here is an example, when we are hungry and want to grab something, and if we hear some sad news, then there is a sudden loss of appetite. Since your mind hears something bad, it signals the gut that the body is not hungry. This means your brain communicates to the gut, and simultaneously the gut communicates to the brain.

There is an entire ecosystem of bacteria and neural networks in our gut. Like we have Central Nervous System (CNS), we have the Enteric Nervous system (ENS) in our gut. ENS is located in the lining of the tissues of the esophagus, stomach, small intestine, and large intestine and makeup of the neurons as CNS. ENS plays a large role in sending information to the brain about what's happening in the gut, which helps control blood flow and other secretions for proper absorption and digestion of the food. The human microbiome has about 100 trillion microbes, mostly live in our gut. [5] The microbiome's primary function is to develop immunity, fight against infections, and provide nutrition to the body so that the gut absorbs more nutrients from the food. 90% of serotonin, our happiness hormone is stored in the gut. But if there is an inflammation in the gut, there is less serotonin secretion, and one will have feelings of sadness and depression. If you are consistently eating processed food, you will produce bacteria that will gain weight. Because of the global food industry, we are becoming more fascinated with it than eating our local food. If we eat what our gut is not supposed to eat, it leads to leaky gut, Inflammatory Bowel Disease (IBD), allergies, inflammation, and other diseases. Due to several factors, our good gut bacteria gets imbalanced. An imbalance in our gut bacteria is known as **dysbiosis.**

There are several factors for this imbalance.

- Over usage of antibiotics is one of the significant factors for dysbiosis. Antibiotics kill bad as well as good bacteria. Broad-spectrum antibiotics can affect 30% of the bacteria in the gut causing a significant drop in diversity. Due to this, there is an alteration in the gut microbiota which causes increased susceptibility to intestinal infections, low immunity [6], and low metabolism. [7]
- Over usage of pain medications. For mild pain, people gulp painkillers regularly, due to which we are disturbing the flora of our gut, causing gastritis and various other ailments. [8]

- High sugar intake, refined flour, processed foods also are major concerns for an imbalance of good gut bacteria. These food increase the growth of fungus and yeast in our body which leads to many diseases. Processed food breaks down into compounds that the harmful bacteria love to eat. After continuous feeding of processed food compounds, these harmful bacteria grow abundantly and cause an unhealthy gut. [9]
- Dysbiosis also occurs due to the consumption of contaminated food. Food contamination causes stomach cramps, nausea, vomiting, diarrhea, and allergies. The most common pathogens that disturb the gut microbiota are E. coli [10] and Salmonella. [11]
- Due to stress. Stress is a significant factor too for causing imbalances of good gut bacteria. Stress may affect brain-gut communication and may cause gut discomfort. Stress is associated with changes in gut bacteria which can influence a person's mood. When stressed, one can eat too much or too little and, there is a tendency that the person ends up eating processed food. Stress can also make the intestinal barrier vulnerable, allowing gut bacteria to enter the body. [12]

Symptoms of dysbiosis

- Gas, bloating, acidity
- Constipation/diarrhea
- Chronic unexplained fatigue
- Bad breath
- Depression, anxiety
- Food allergies and sensitivities
- Acne, Eczema, and other skin problems
- Rise in candida and other fungal infections
- Asthma and other breathing problems
- Headache, memory loss, confusion
- All types of arthritis

A body's health depends on a healthy gut, and many diseases arise due to wrong gut bacteria. Patients with IBD have decreased bacterial diversity as compared to healthy individuals. Even skin diseases, allergies, asthma, arthritis, and some neurological disorders are due to the lack of a particular bacteria. If you are feeling down or gloomy, most of the time, it could be a sign that your microbiome is not healthy. Our gut microbiota plays a vital role in our health physically, psychologically, and emotionally. Clinically it is proven that when you add good bacteria to your diet, there are fewer chances of contracting these diseases.

Every person's microbiota is unique; if some food suits one, it doesn't mean that it will suit all. Listen to your body and incorporate new food one at a time and see if it's giving any positive or negative effects.

Now the question is how to keep the gut flora healthy. Here are some ways to keep your gut healthy.

- Eat your traditional staple food. Eat whatever your Grandma used to eat.
- Go for locally grown seasonal organic produce.
- Eat fermented foods like Curd, Kanji, Fermented rice, Kefir, Sauerkraut as these foods contain live bacteria that benefit our gut. Eat more prebiotics and probiotics. [13]
- Have more buttermilk and lassi.
- Include collagen in your diet as it regulates the stomach acid secretion, repairs the stomach lining, heals leaky gut, and strengthens the gut.
- Keep antibiotic use to a minimum. Don't take antibiotics for simple cold and viral infections, and look out for natural home remedies.
- Reduce the intake of sugar and artificial sweeteners.
- Add more fiber and leafy vegetables.

- Incorporate more carminative spices [14] like ginger, cumin, fennel, caraway. [15]
- Include pickles in your meal. When food items are pickled, their antioxidant powers are enhanced. Eat pickles in small quantities, do not overeat them. Make pickles at home as store-bought pickles have preservatives and additives. If you suffer from high blood pressure, ulcers, heart disease, then pickles are not for you.
- Reduce stress – By doing yoga and meditation, we can lower the stress hormone, which positively affects gut bacteria.
- Exercise combined with healthy eating produces more good gut bacteria.

Probiotics are living microorganisms that can be consumed through curd and fermented foods. If we have a healthy gut, our body works perfectly. They are good bacteria that provide health benefits. When there is an imbalance in gut bacteria, it results in various diseases. [16]

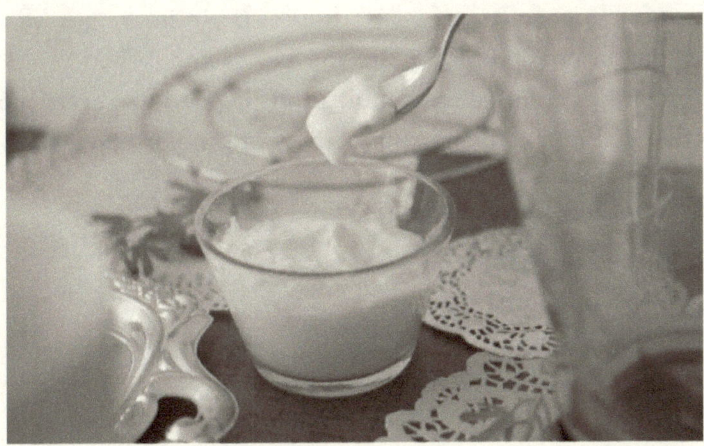

Picture 4: Curd

Probiotics help in good digestion and help in reducing inflammation, allergies, eczema. It plays a fundamental role in preserving health. It also boosts the immune system and improves overall health. You can get probiotics from curd, Indian Kanji, fermented foods like kefir, sauerkraut, sourdough bread, etc. When we ferment the food, essential nutrients are released into the body, making us healthier. Lactobacillus and Bifidobacterium species are the most common and beneficial bacteria.

Prebiotics act as food for probiotics. Prebiotics boosts probiotic function. It is a type of non-digestible fiber. It acts as a fertilizer for the good bacteria already present. Prebiotics works with probiotics to allow some positive changes in the gastrointestinal tract. A high diet of prebiotics helps in reducing the risk of colon cancer. It increases calcium absorption. Fiber is the source of prebiotics, and foods high in fiber are prebiotic. Garlic, onions, bananas, raw honey, whole wheat, barley, oats, apple, flaxseeds, chickpeas act as a prebiotic. [17]

In Ayurveda, we believe that all diseases arise because of poor digestion and poor absorption of food. Even the father of modern medicine, Hippocrates, said: "All diseases begin in the gut." So, for better gut health, probiotics are the key factor. When probiotics and prebiotics are used in combination, it provides several health benefits. Prebiotics enhances the activity of probiotics.

Benefits of probiotics and prebiotics

- Improved digestion
- Reduces inflammation
- Better gut health
- Healthy cholesterol levels
- Helps in weight loss
- Regulates hormone levels
- Helps in IBS
- Treats leaky gut syndrome

- It helps in improving skin problems like eczema, psoriasis
- Prevents and treats enteric infections

Leaky gut syndrome We have a barrier between our gut and the bloodstream to prevent harmful substances from entering the bloodstream. In a leaky gut, these junctions loosen up, and harmful substances enter the bloodstream causing inflammation, resulting in various diseases [18].

There is a connection between the gut, brain, and skin. If digestion is poor, an overgrowth of unhealthy bacteria causes inflammation, which can manifest in the brain or skin, causing various diseases. Symptoms of leaky gut are gas, bloating, acidity, IBS, allergies, inflammation, hormonal imbalance, eczema, arthritis.

What causes a leaky gut? Bad food habits, medications, toxins, stress, etc. Sugar, gluten, dairy products, white flour are the major culprits. Fungal or bacterial overgrowth also causes a leaky gut. Pain medications, antibiotics, steroids also add to this syndrome.

How to heal a leaky gut Eliminate all food items that cause leaky gut like sugar, gluten, dairy. Eliminate one food at a time and see how you feel. Make a food journal. Check what food causes digestive issues or other problems. Remove that food from your diet. Eat your food slowly and chew well. As digestion starts in the mouth, it is essential to chew well to generate more digestive enzymes. Look at your food and enjoy the color and aroma. If you are under stress, do not eat; wait till you calm down.

Reduce the usage of NSAIDs (non-steroidal anti-inflammatory drugs). Eat wholesome foods like fresh seasonal fruits and vegetables. Take lots of fiber-rich foods. Incorporate more Omega-3- fatty acids like flaxseeds, walnuts, pumpkin seeds, sunflower seeds, fish. Take more probiotics and prebiotics. Have cultured dairy products like curd, buttermilk, and Greek yogurt.

Postbiotics are the byproducts of probiotic metabolism. When dietary fiber breaks down and ferments in the colon into several products, we call them postbiotics. Postbiotics are the alternative to maintaining digestive health. Examples are curd with live bacteria, kefir, dark chocolate, pickles [19].

Here are a few healthy and easy-to-make recipes of fermented food to increase the good gut bacteria.

Kanji is a fermented probiotic drink to improve digestion.

Carrot Kanji

Prep: 15 mins; Cook: Nil

Ingredients

- 3 purple carrots (If you don't get purple carrots, use the regular red or orange carrots)
- 1 beetroot
- 3-4 cups water
- 1 tbsp mustard powder
- ½ tsp black rock salt

Method

- Peel the carrots and the beetroot.
- Cut into cubes.
- Mix all the ingredients in a glass jar.
- Cover the lid and let stand in the Sun for 3-4 days.
- Keep shaking the jar everyday 2-3 times.
- After 4 days, you can drink and store the rest of it in the refrigerator.
- You can strain the mix and chew the carrots and beets.

Kanji improves digestion, boosts immunity, and is good for the eyes and heart.

Buttermilk

Prep: 5 mins; Cook: Nil

Ingredients

- 2 tbsp plain curd
- 1 cup water
- ¼ tsp roasted cumin powder
- 1 small piece of ginger
- 1 pinch of rock salt

Method

- Mix all the ingredients in a jar and shake well.
- Drink at room temperature.

It improves digestion, boosts appetite, maintains strong bones and teeth, lowers cholesterol. In Ayurveda, Buttermilk is called "Takra." Buttermilk is very helpful in increasing good gut bacteria and helps ward off many diseases, including IBS.

Fermented Rice Gruel

Prep: 20 mins; Cook: 15

Ingredients

- 1 cup rice

- 5 cups water for boiling
- 2 glasses of buttermilk
- 2-3 Bird's eye chilies

Method

- Boil rice in an open pot.
- Once the rice is soft, remove it from the stove. Drain excess water.
- Allow rice to cool to room temperature.
- Add buttermilk and chilies to the cooked rice and store them in a clay pot.
- Leave the pot overnight.
- The rice would ferment the next morning.

In this way, nutrients from rice are densely available, and the nutritional value increases. This rice gives a cooling effect to the body.

Sauerkraut

Prep: 5 mins; Cook: Nil

Ingredients

- 1 small cabbage
- 1 shredded carrot
- 2 tbsp sea salt
- ½ tbsp caraway seeds

Method

- Thinly slice the organic cabbage.

- In a large bowl, mix cabbage, shredded carrot, caraway seeds, and salt.
- Mix it well and let it stand for few minutes.
- Transfer the cabbage mixture into a glass container.
- Leave this mixture for 3-4 weeks in a dark and cool area.
- Post 3-4 weeks refrigerator for usage.
- You can use this mixture in wraps, sandwiches, or as a side dish with your meals.

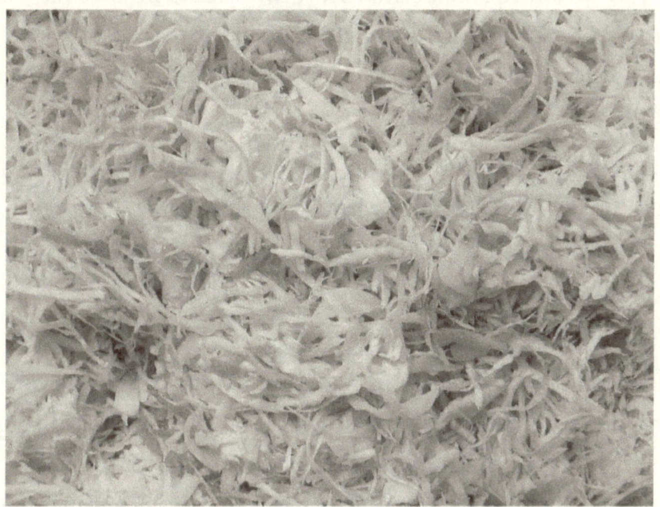

Picture 5: Sauerkraut

How probiotics and prebiotics are good for athletes

Probiotics help athletes maintain good health so that they can train better and perform well. Probiotics are important for athletes to aid better digestion and absorption of food. A healthy gut can absorb nutrients from the food better, which is important for an athlete who needs to get nutrients from a wholesome diet. Moreover, athletes have an overall active lifestyle. Due to the high demands of training sessions and events, there is more strain on the digestive system. It's a wise idea to incorporate fermented food regularly.

An upset stomach during a run is a common problem. Overtraining also leads to stomach issues. If you incorporate probiotics and prebiotics in your diet plan, good gut bacteria levels increase and thus can ease the symptoms of stomach distress.

Probiotics can also help in reducing inflammation in muscles. If you take probiotics consistently, it minimizes muscle damage. So, probiotics are key to improve athletic performance and recovery. It also reduces the number of sick days as probiotics prevent the growth of harmful bacteria.

Including probiotics in the diet is a great way to get healthy bacteria and easily eliminate waste products.

Gut cleansing

We feel like we have emptied the intestines; however, some undigested particles still get stuck to the intestinal lining and stomach. These undigested particles create toxins in the body which is the major cause of various diseases. There are various methods through which we can cleanse the stomach like Vaman dhauti, enema. These are the most important parts of panchakarma therapy in Ayurveda.

Vaman Dhauti and **Kunjal Kriya** is a purification technique to wash out toxins and undigested food particles from the stomach lining through the mouth. Vaman means "To Vomit."

Process of Vaman Dhauti

Prepare saline water by dissolving 2 teaspoons of salt in a litre of warm water. Sit in a squatted position and drink this water to your full capacity. Usually, we drink water slowly; however, for Vaman dhauti, it should be gulped fast so that one feels nauseous and can vomit. Expanding and contracting abdominal muscles aids in the process. Bend forward down and insert two fingers into your throat; this will cause vomiting reflux. In the process of Vaman dhauti, undigested food particles get eliminated. Once the water comes out entirely, then wash your mouth and face. Relax in Shavasana for 10 minutes. This is also called washing the alimentary canal.

Benefits

- It cleanses the esophagus and stomach and clears out all the undigested food.
- It removes extra mucus from the upper respiratory tract and relieves the symptoms of bronchitis, sore throat, cough with phlegm, asthma, and other upper respiratory ailments.
- It helps in indigestion, acidity, and gas problem. It increases digestive fire.
- According to Ayurveda, it balances the Kapha-pitta doshas in the stomach.

Precautions

- It's an easy practice to be done at home; however, first-timers can do it under guidance.
- It should not be performed if you have ulcers, stomach hernia, or other stomach and esophagus-related problems.
- Vaman dhauti should not be done if someone is suffering from heart disease or high blood pressure.
- Should not be performed by pregnant or nursing mothers.

The difference between Vaman dhauti and Kunjal Kriya is that Kunjal kriya is performed on an empty stomach, and Vaman dhauti can be performed after 3-4 hours of having a meal.

Basti Karma (Enema) This is one of the main procedures of Panchkarma. This has preventive and curative perspectives. In Basti, the medicated oils or herbal decoctions are administered through the anus.

There are several types of Basti; however, we shall not dwell deep into it. Some people perform enema at home with a very simple solution of salt and water.

Benefits

- Highly beneficial in cleansing the colon.
- Balances all the Doshas, particularly Vata dosha.
- Relieves constipation
- Helps in many Vata-related disorders like arthritis and gout.
- Promotes longevity.

Precautions

- Basti should not be performed if the person is suffering from rectum bleeding, diarrhea, asthma, tuberculosis, emaciation.
- Advise performing under medical supervision.

Ayurveda

*"This 5000-year-old knowledge of science of life is
our doorway to a healthy and blissful life. Everyone
should incorporate its teachings every single day in our life."*

Ayurveda [20] is the ancient Indian system of medicine. It is a 5000-year-old system. Ayurveda is made up of two components- "Ayur" and "Veda." "Ayur" means life, and "Veda" means science. Ayurveda is "The science of life." Ayurveda considers a holistic and simple form of the healing approach.

The two most important aims of Ayurveda are

- Swasthyas Swasthya rakshanam- to protect the health of healthy people
- Aturasya Vikar Prashamanamcha- to cure diseases of sick people

Everything in the world is made up of five elements, including the human body. These five elements called "Panchamahabhuta" are Air, Fire, Water, Ether, and Earth. The food we eat, weather, etc., are examples of the presence of these elements. The knowledge of Ayurveda has its written origins in the Vedas. The Vedas were written back in 2500 BC or earlier. Ayurveda is considered the "upveda" to the Atharva Veda. Atharva Veda is the first medical textbook and is the fourth book of the Vedas. The Rigveda contains series of prescriptions that can help humans overcome various ailments. The

Charaka Samhita and Sushruta Samhita are the two foundational texts of this field.

Ayurveda has a different approach to diagnose illnesses. Different ways to diagnose diseases are checking pulse, tongue, vision, touch, speech, urine, stool, and appearance.

Ayurveda addresses all aspects of life. Prevention and treatment emphasize changing the diet, lifestyle modifications, and the use of herbs.

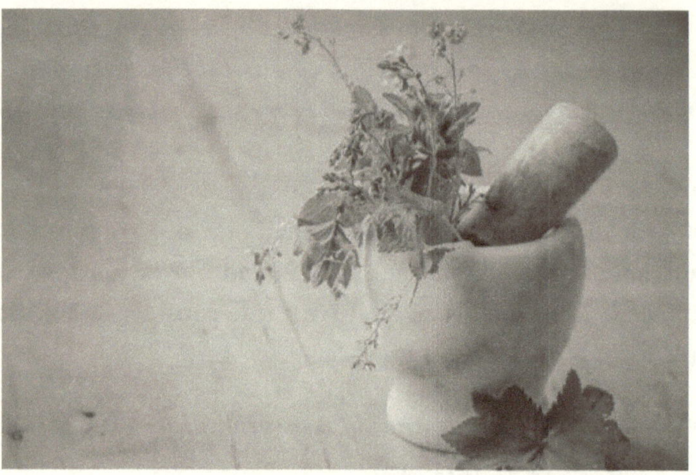

Picture 6: Stone Mortar & Pestle

Panchbhootas (five elements) According to Ayurveda, panchbhootas are the basis of all cosmic creation. All living organisms on Earth are made of these five elements.

Earth (Prithvi)- This element represents the solid state of matter. Bones, teeth, tissues are considered earth elements.

Water (Jal)- It represents the liquid state. Our blood, lymph, other fluids are made up of water.

Fire (Agni)- It is responsible for digestion, absorption, and assimilation. Fire transforms food into energy.

Air (Vayu)- It represents the gaseous state of matter. It is the key element required for fire to burn. It represents movement, contraction.

Ether (Aakash)- Represents the space. A sense of ether element is hearing.

These five elements combine in different ways in humans to govern body, mind, and spirit.

Ayurvedic body types

According to Ayurveda, each one of us has a unique mix of three-body constitutions. These three constitutions are called Doshas.

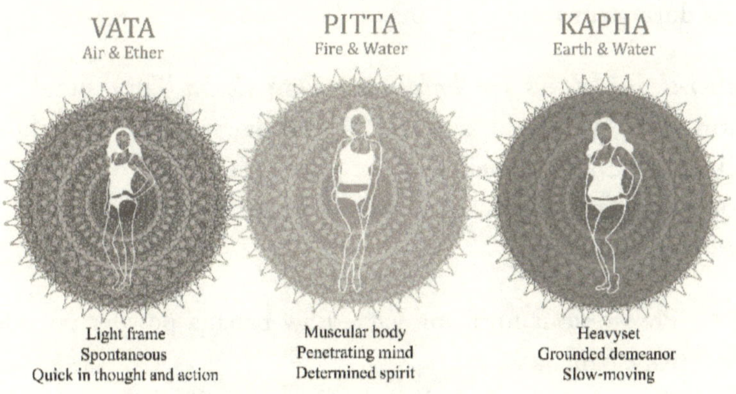

Picture 7: Vata Pitta Kapha

There are three Doshas in our body

- Vata

- Pitta
- Kapha

Each individual has its unique proportion of these Doshas that shapes our nature and health. For each element, there are balanced and imbalanced expressions. So as long as these three Doshas remain in balance, the system digests food properly and growth and development follow their natural course. If there is a disturbance of any one of these elements, the system becomes imbalanced, and pain and diseases are inevitable. This imbalance alters body chemistry and reduces the effectiveness of the system's natural defense. Eat food as per your Doshas type. If Vata is aggravated, eat food to pacify Vata.

Vata: Qualities reflects the elements of Space and Air. It acts as a carrier; Vayu can carry anything. Vata people are generally thin, very active but get tired easily. Vata people have dry skin and hair and often suffer from constipation, arthritis, cracked lips, and heels. They do not like sitting idle and are always on the move. Athletes who have increased Vata property think too much, feel nervous, feel dizzy during runs and get pains easily.

General guidelines for balancing Vata dosha They should eat warm food. Avoid cold, dry, and hard-to-digest foods. They should include good fats in their diet like ghee, nuts, seeds, and coconut. Dry, astringent, bitter tastes should be avoided. Concentrate on breathing exercises.

- Pre-workout meal for Vata- Raw banana powder porridge/ Ripe banana
- Post-workout meal- Paneer/Almond milk chia seeds drink/ Scrambled eggs

Pitta: Qualities that reflect the elements of Fire and Water. Pitta originates in the stomach. Digestion and metabolism are the two main processes of Pitta. Pitta is a thin and hot fluid. Pitta people usually have a good digestive fire. They cannot tolerate heat and often suffer from acidity, jaundice, bleeding gums, ulcers, anger and frustration. Pitta dominant athletes also sweat profusely.

General guidelines to balance Pitta dosha They should avoid excessive heat and eat cooling foods like cucumber, kokum, watermelon, coconut water, rose syrup, mulethi. Care should be taken to avoid very hot and spicy foods. Salt should also be taken with restriction. Cold showers help people with pitta dosha.

- Pre-workout food for Pitta- Boiled Sweet potato/Boiled Potato/Curd + banana + honey
- Post-workout food- Curd rice/Nutty coconut foxtail

Kapha: Qualities reflecting the elements of Earth and Water. Kapha is white, smooth, sticky, cold, and sweet fluid. Kapha dominant people are usually heavy, cool, and slow. Their skin and hair are oily and smooth. They have a glow on their faces. They love sitting and sleeping. They also show signs of slow digestion. They have sluggish bowels and suffer frequent candida infections.

Kapha athletes are consistent in their runs and have a calm mind but are sometimes too lazy for training runs. They enjoy big meals and feel lethargic.

General guidelines to balance Kapha dosha: Eat light, warm foods. Avoid oily, deep-fried food. Use warm spices like ginger, black pepper, garlic, onions. Stay more active.

- Pre-workout food for Kapha- Bread with honey/Oats
- Post-workout- Sprouts salad/Chickpea salad/Boiled eggs

Indians usually have a dominance of Vata and Pitta in men and Pitta in women. Eat food as per your body constitution.

Below is the **Doshas Table,** which helps determine one's Ayurvedic body type. You can have one dominant or two prominent Doshas. Once you know your Doshas, you can balance the body with food choices.

Physical	Vata	Pitta	Kapha
Body Size	Tall & Thin/ Short & Thin	Average	Tall & Stocky/ Short & Stocky
Bodyweight	Below average. Difficulty putting on weight	Moderate, no difficulties in gaining or losing weight	Heavy difficulty in losing weight
Skin	Dry, thin, rough, cool to touch	Soft, acne, moles, warm to touch	Oily, moist, greasy, glowing
Hair	Dry, coarse, brittle	Oily, straight, greying, balding	Thick, oily, curly, luxurious
Eyes	Small, dry, sunken, blink a lot	Medium size, sharp gaze	Big, round, calm gaze, eyes puffiness
Lips	Dry, chapped, cracked	Soft and pink	Large, full, smooth
Nails	Dry, rough, brittle	Pink, shiny	Thick, smooth, strong
Teeth	Crooked, uneven, receding gums	Even, yellowish, gums bleed easily	Large, even, gleaming teeth
Appetite	Irregular, variable	Very strong, cannot skip meals	Constant, tolerate hunger
Digestion	Irregular, gaseous, bloating	Quick, heartburn	Slow digestion and metabolism
Bowel movement	Irregular, constipated	Loose, soft, burning	Slow, thick stool with mucous
Sleep	Irregular, less, awakes easily	Sound	Long, sound, find it difficult to wake up

Physical	**Vata**	**Pitta**	**Kapha**
Walk	Fast, short steps	Moderate, Long steps	Slow, gracefully
Endurance	Low energy comes in spurts, then get tired easily, can't push too hard	Moderate/high, can push too hard	Very good, high endurance and stamina
Pace of activity	Fast, hyperactive	Medium speed/ intense	Slow, steady
Perspiration	Scanty with no odor	Heavy with a strong odor	Moderate or heavy with no odor
Speech	Fast, talkative	Précised, well organized	Slow and calm
Voice	High pitched, fast, weeping	Medium, tone, sharp, laughing	Low, slow-paced, pleasant with moments of silence
Memory	Short term	Average	Excellent long-term memory hardly forgets
Weather preference	Likes warm, dislikes windy, dry, and cold days	Likes cool dislikes heat	Likes warm, dry, dislikes cold and rain
Lifestyle	Highly active	Active	Rather inactive
Taste preference	Sweet, sour, salty	Sweet, bitter, astringent	Bitter, pungent, astringent
Thirst	Variable	Always thirsty	Sparse need for water
Mood	Mood changes quickly	Intense emotions	Steady emotions
Mental tendencies	To ask and theorize	To judge	To be stable and logical
I love	Art, travel	Sports, politics, luxuries	Good food

Physical	Vata	Pitta	Kapha
Decisions	Decision making is problematic	Makes decisions quickly and determined	Decides after thinking thoroughly
Financial	Buy on impulse, wasteful	Spends money lavishly	Good at saving money
Friendship	Knows a lot of people but has few friends	Friends are more work-related, changes with job	Loyal with many friends
Consider me as	Lively, intuitive	Motivated, warm, perceptive	Resilient, loyal
Your acquaintances describe you as	Enthusiastic, changeable	Friendly, independent	Relaxed, deliberate
Thinking style	Restless, quick	Organized, efficient	Slow, methodical
Creativity level	Full of ideas, but cannot follow	Inventive, good to follow ideas	Best in fields of business
I process information	Quickly	Medium speed	Slowly
Most sensitive to	Noise	Bright light	Strong odors
I like to learn new things best by	Listening to the speaker	Reading	Associating it with another memory
Emotionally	Worry, anxiety, moody, emotional	Angry, irritated	Stay calm

Table 1

Six tastes of Ayurveda: Ayurveda recommends including all these six tastes in every meal so that one can have balanced nutrition and good health. When Doshas are imbalanced, these six tastes help to maintain them in a balanced state. By including all these tastes in your diet, one will not crave junk food. Each taste affects tridoshas.

Sweet (Madhura) Sweet taste consists of water and Earth.

This taste is good for balancing Vata and Pitta. It increases Kapha. For people with lean bodies and those who need to gain weight, emphasis can be given to sweet taste. It nourishes male and female reproductive systems. Sweet taste, as per Ayurvedic six tastes, does not mean processed sugar. It means the food when eaten, leaves some light sweet taste on the tongue. Examples are wheat, rice, dates, licorice root, pumpkins, sweet potato, ghee, butter, coconut, and jaggery.

Sour (Amala) Sour taste consists of water and fire.

This taste improves appetite and digestion. It decreases Vata. Examples are lemon, vinegar, fermented food, pickles, tamarind.

Salty (Lavana) Salty taste consists of Earth and fire.

It stimulates digestion, helps in absorbing the nutrients. It acts as a laxative. Examples are Himalayan pink salt, sea salt, and sea vegetables.

Pungent (Katu) Pungent taste consists of air and fire.

It is considered the hottest food. It helps in digestion and clearing sinuses. It also helps in dissolving the extra fat in the body. Pungent foods are penetrative and detoxify the body. It is good for Kapha people. Examples are ginger, garlic, onions, hot spices, radish, cinnamon, etc.

Bitter (Tikta) Bitter taste consists of air and ether.

It has a cooling effect on the human body and is good for Pitta and Kapha people. Examples are green vegetables, herbal teas, turmeric, fenugreek, bitter melon, etc.

Indian gooseberry (Amla) is the only food that has five tastes except for salty taste. Do include amla in your diet.

Astringent (Kashaya) Astringent taste consists of air and Earth.

Pitta people benefit from eating astringent foods. These foods have anti-diarrheal properties. Examples are Pomegranates, green beans, unripe fruits.

In a nutshell, for Vata disorders, use salty, sour, and sweet tastes food.

For pitta disorders, one should consume bitter, sweet, and astringent foods.

For Kapha, disorders consume pungent, bitter, and astringent foods.

Types of food as per Ayurveda

- Sattvic
- Rajasic
- Tamasic

Sattvic Diet consists of fresh, organic fruits, vegetables, nuts, seeds, whole grains, beans, lentils, dairy products, cold-pressed oils, and some spices. Sattva means life, so eat food that is freshly prepared. Sattvic food digests easily and provides energy to the body. Such food refreshes and rejuvenates the body. A sattvic diet also follows Ahimsa, which is the practice of non-violence. Sattvic food gives more clarity and the quality of forgiveness. Khichdi is a perfect example of sattvic food.

Importance of Khichdi in Ayurveda

Khichdi is a traditional Indian food prepared for thousands of years. Khichdi can balance all three Doshas. It is known as tridoshic food. So, whatever your Prakriti is, khichdi fits in all. It is light, nourishing, and restorative. It heals various diseases. It is easy on digestion hence used in cleansing therapy in Ayurveda. It is high in dietary fiber. When we combine dal and rice, it is a good source of complete protein. People who are gluten insensitive can also have khichdi. It is also used as a weaning food to nourish babies.

Khichdi

Prep: 1 hr 25 mins; Cook: 25 mins

Ingredients

- ½ cup moong dal
- ¾ cup basmati rice
- 1tsp cumin
- 2tsp ghee
- Chopped ginger
- ½ tsp turmeric
- Salt to taste
- 5-6 cups water

Method

- Rinse rice and dal several times, then soak it for an hour.
- Drain the water.
- In a pan, add ghee and cumin seeds. Let it splutter, then add ginger, saute it.
- Add rice, dal, turmeric powder, salt, and water. Mix it and cover the pan.
- Boil it and reduce the heat. Let it simmer until it gets soft and fluffy.

This is the general recipe of khichdi; however, you can attempt variations as per Doshas. For pacifying Vata, temper the khichdi with asafetida and homemade/organic cow ghee. For pacifying Pitta add coriander, cinnamon in the above recipe. For pacifying Kapha add black pepper and dry ginger powder.

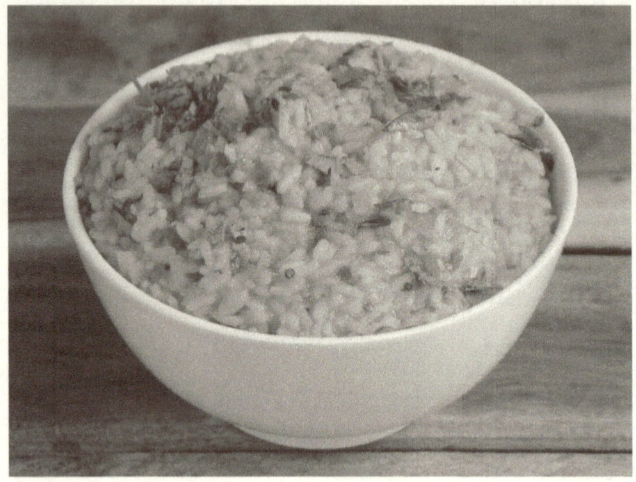

Picture 8: Kichadi

Rajasic food has a stimulating effect on the body. All tempting foods come under this category. Examples are tea, coffee, colas, chocolates, fried food. This palette leads to irritability in the mind and body.

Tamasic All processed foods come under this category, like white flour, excess sugary foods, preservative-laden foods, bakery products, meat, alcohol, and stale food. When we microwave food, that food also turns tamasic. Tamasic food does not have any nutrient value and is highly acidic. These foods are very difficult to digest and produce sluggishness in the body. Tamasic diet does not nourish the brain nor the body. All cooked food becomes tamasic after 3 hours of cooking, according to Bhagavad Gita. [21]

It is recommended to follow a sattvic diet, but some rajasic and tamasic food may be introduced to the diet depending on the physical work.

Incompatible foods (Virudh Aahar)

When different food substances of different taste, energy, and post-digestive effect are combined, the digestive fire gets overloaded and produces toxins. We feel good or bad depending on the food combinations we eat. As per Ayurveda, certain food combinations should be avoided. The poor combining of food results in indigestion, gastric reflux, gas bloating, allergies, colds, congestion, skin diseases, and weight gain.

Incompatible foods as per Ayurveda [22]

- Milk and fruits should never be combined. A lot of people enjoy their mango or other fruit shakes, but that's a bad idea. Fruits must be eaten alone. Do not mix with milk.
- Dairy with meat/fish should not be taken together. Milk is a coolant, and meat has hot potency. It is hard on digestion.
- Ghee and honey should not be mixed in equal quantities.
- Honey should never be cooked. Cooked honey produces toxins.
- Sweet and sour fruits should not be eaten together.
- Radish with milk is highly incompatible

Do take care of food combinations while eating. [23]

Some foods should not be eaten in a particular season or time of the day, like curd should not be consumed at night. The best time to consume curd and buttermilk is at lunch. Avoid cold water during or after meals. Have fruits during the daytime, especially empty stomach or in between two meals.

Health

In 1946, the World Health Organization defined health as "a state of complete physical, mental and social well-being and not merely the absence of disease." The food we eat affects all three aspects of our health. Eating well is vital for a healthy and active life. Fill your plate with colors of the rainbow by choosing a variety of colored vegetables that enhances health.

State of Mind

It is important to eat a balanced diet with a calm mind to improve digestion. How you feel when you eat also matters. If you are angry, sad, irritated, upset, do not eat your food at that time. Your body will not digest it properly, and nutrients won't get absorbed optimally. As our mental state and digestive system influence each other, it is best to wait until the mind calms down and then have food for better digestion and absorption. We should be conscious of our eating.

Even the person who cooks the food should be in a calm and happy state of mind. If you serve and eat food with love and care, then you are getting the right food.

Eat Mindfully

Multitasking is not a good idea while eating. Concentrate on your food and eat slow. Enjoy the color, aroma, flavor, and texture. Take small bites and chew well. Since digestion of food starts in the mouth, it is essential to chew well to release more digestive enzymes for better digestion. The body sends a satiation signal after 20 minutes when one starts eating. Chew the food until it liquefies and then swallows. Eat only when hungry. When eating, concentrate on only eating with no distraction via mobile, newspaper, television, etc. Mindful eating helps to gain control over eating habits.

Nowadays, people grab breakfast on their way to work and eat in such a way that they want only to fill their stomachs. During lunch, they eat at their desk while working on their laptop. They think they are eating, but this is mindless eating. Mindless eating means not paying attention while eating, which leads to gas, bloating, acidity, overeating, weight gain, and many more diseases. When we are distracted, it is hard for the body to listen to signals about food. We cannot differentiate between emotional or true hunger. Give mindful eating a try to see the difference.

The concept of "Ama": When we eat food, it should digest fully and get absorbed properly, and then expel out of the body as waste products. However, it does not always happen that way. Due to inappropriate eating habits, stress, inactivity, pollution, and mindless eating, food absorption and assimilation are hampered. It results in undigested food. This undigested food is named "AMA" (toxins). Ama is a Sanskrit word that means undigested, unripe. This Ama is heavy, sticky, foul-smelling. Ayurveda believes Ama is said to be the root cause of all the diseases occurring in the body. Depending upon where the ama is in the body, it can cause a thick coating on the tongue, poor circulation, gastric issues, weight gain, inflammation, and many more diseases. Strong digestive fire or Agni is essential to maintain optimal health. When digestion and metabolism are good, food eaten gets digested well. For poor digestion, it is apt to use digestive spices like ginger, fennel, black pepper, carom seeds, cumin seeds, and pippali. Practice regular exercise, steam bath, detoxification, and fast to help get rid of Ama.

Why fresh food is better than refrigerated or microwaved food

Nowadays, people cook food in large portions and store it in the refrigerator and consume it for the next 3-4 days or more. Refrigerating or freezing lowers the enzyme activity, which is essential for digestion and nutrient absorption. As per Ayurveda, eating leftover food is not recommended as it is considered tamasic food, which is not suitable to eat. Moreover, it loses nutritional value and also can add digestive problems. Long ago, when there were no refrigerators, people used to buy fresh produce and cook fresh every day. Today it is an effort to make fresh food for every meal, but that's worth it. When food is reheated in a microwave, the food gets tamasic. When food stored in plastic containers is reheated in the microwave, certain chemicals leach into the food, which leads to several health problems. That food, if eaten, weakens the immune system. When we use a microwave, we are exposing ourselves to radiation. These radiations accumulate over time and affect the frequencies of the brain. It leads to a negative impact on the brain and the human body. Nothing is more important than a healthy body, so it is advisable to avoid microwaving the food and start making fresh food for every meal.

Natural urges we shouldn't be suppressing

Ayurveda suggests that one should not hold natural urges. When urges are suppressed, it interferes with the body's state of balance. There are 13 natural urges which should not be suppressed - Sneeze, Sleep, Cough, Cry, Yawn, Hunger, Burp, Fart, Vomit, Thirst, Heavy or Fast breathing after exertion, Urination, and defecate. If one happens to suppress these urges regularly, it may arise as a disease sooner or later. The body needs to keep itself in a healthy condition. So, the body needs detoxification regularly. By suppressing these thirteen urges, we interfere with the smooth functioning of the body.

There are some urges we need to suppress.

- Anger
- Greed
- Jealousy
- Hatred
- Envy

Dinacharya [24] means daily routine. If we follow the daily routine as per Ayurveda, we can lead a healthy, happy, and full of energy lifestyle. Dinacharya balances the Doshas. It improves the quality of life and promotes longevity. Everyone should follow a daily routine.

- Waking up early in the morning is the first routine everyone should follow. Waking up an hour and a half to two hours before sunrise is the best time as the air is fresh and pure. This time is called "Bramamuhurat." This is the time of the day when nature releases the highest amount of pure and clean oxygen.
- Drink two-three glasses of warm water. Beginners can start with one glass and gradually increase the intake.
- Clear the urinary bladder and bowel. One should not hold these natural urges, which give way to many diseases.
- Wash face, nose, and eyes. Fill the mouth with water and hold this water for few seconds before spitting it out and then splash water on the eyes.
- Brush teeth and scrape the tongue.
- Oil pulling: [25] A lot of diseases originate from the oral cavity. Oil pulling helps clean the oral cavity and reduces the chances of infection. Method for Oil Pulling – Take a tablespoon of coconut oil and swish it inside the mouth for 15-20 minutes. Once done, rinse the mouth with warm water. Oil pulling is good for teeth, gums, and overall oral health.
- Do your workouts.
- Garshana: (Dry Brushing) Dry brushing means brushing the skin with a dry brush. The skin is typically brushed toward the heart. Pay attention to your lymph nodes while doing dry brushing. It's good for stimulating lymphatic flow, as the lymphatic system is a major part of the body's immune

system. It also removes dead skin. It also greatly helps to reduce cellulite. Choose the natural bristle brush with a handle. Dry brushing can be done before showering.

- Oil Massage: Nothing soothes a stressed mind and body as much as a massage does. Regular massage keeps the body working optimally. Regular massage soothes the muscles, aids in proper blood circulation, and thereby heal sore muscles. It lubricates the joints and helps in reducing the symptoms of arthritis, and relaxes the mind. We should always massage towards the direction of the heart. Several oils can be used for massages like sesame oil, coconut oil, mustard oil, and olive oil.

- Take a shower.

- Meditate and pray.

- Eat a home-cooked nutritious breakfast.

- You are all set to go for your work and daily chores.

- Lunch should be taken between 12 to 2 pm. As Pitta is high during lunchtime, it should be the largest meal of the day.

- Have an early and light dinner. It should be between 6 to 7 pm as digestion is low at this time, so best to opt for a light dinner.

- Strolling is important after dinner to stimulate digestion.

- Oil in the naval- Before sleeping, put 3-4 drops of oil in the naval and massage the surrounding area. Several oils can be used, like mustard oil, coconut oil, almond oil, neem oil, and ghee. One can choose an oil depending on their health and the health issues one needs to address. If pimples and acne need attention, it is good to use neem oil. For cracked lips or stomach pain, mustard oil is the best. For dryness of the eyes coconut oil is recommended.

- Relax your body, take deep breaths and sleep well. Try to sleep at the same time every night

Most of us pay attention to healthy eating and exercising. However, we don't pay much attention to our sleeping habits. Good sleep repairs and rejuvenates the body and has a relaxing effect on the heart and blood vessels. Healthy sleep enhances well-being. Athletes should be more cautious about their sleeping habits, as it impacts their performance. Insufficient sleep leads to fatigue and makes athletes prone to injury. Moreover, sleep is essential for muscle recovery.

Tips for good sleep

- Sleep at the same time every night
- Have an early dinner.
- Restrict caffeine intake after 4 pm as caffeine disrupts the sleep cycle.
- Have a warm shower before hitting the bed and finish off by pouring a mug of warm water mixed with a spoon of Epsom salt.
- Let go of your thoughts. Pray and meditate.
- One can have a glass of warm milk with nutmeg and almonds.
- Chamomile tea stimulates sleep.
- Get a foot and head massage using oil as per one's doshas.
- Try Yog Nidra [26], a form of yogic sleep that relaxes one's mind and aids sound sleep.
- Ashwagandha with warm milk helps people with sleep disorders.
- Other ayurvedic herbs that can be used for insomnia are Jatamansi, Brahmi, Shankhpushpi, Vacha. These herbs can be taken under the supervision of an Ayurvedic practitioner.

A self-care daily routine is necessary for the well-being of the body and mind and also for optimum performance in running events. Only healthy bodies can perform well, so it is important to incorporate the Ayurvedic dincharya.

Ayurveda believes in digestive power. If digestion is strong, food can be digested and absorbed properly, and organs stay nourished. But if the digestive fire or Agni is low, one may suffer from many ailments. With inadequate digestion, bad bacteria multiply faster on the unabsorbed food leading to fermentation which causes several digestive issues. When food is not digested, nutrients aren't absorbed by the body too. Skin health, inflammation, pains, mood, anger depends upon good digestion. One can have better digestion by following Ayurvedic Dincharaya and by inculcating some home remedies. Firstly never overeat, listen to your stomach and stop eating when you get the first sign of fullness. Secondly, chew ginger slices before eating meals or have Curcuma manga (Mango-ginger) pickle during meals. Do follow the mindful eating practice. Take small bites and chew 32 times. Swallow only when food liquifies so that digestive enzymes release into the mouth and stomach, yielding better digestion. As per Ayurveda, lunch should be the biggest and heaviest meal of the day. This is because, at that time, the digestive fire in a body is strong. This is also called the pitta period, and if one eats a good, healthy big meal, it will digest well. Undigested food results in many health issues, including weight gain. Our body works according to the Sun's movement, and our digestive fire is high when Sun is strongest. So, when the Sun goes down, food portions should be small. These guidelines are for those who are healthy and leading a normal lifestyle, but few guidelines are altered depending on the health condition of an individual.

Protocol to follow before every meal [27]

- *Warm-up the body*, Take slow long deep breaths. Expand the abdomen as you inhale and relax as you exhale. Do "Bhastrika pranayama" for 30 seconds, then again deep abdominal breathing.
- *Massage your ears to cut cravings*, as there are many pressure points in the ear.

- Before starting the meal, have freshly grated ginger with some rock salt and lemon and chew well.
- *Avoid water* along with your meals but if required, have few sips of warm water.
- *Chew well* and eat slow.
- Few minutes post eating, massage the left side of your rib cage.
- Drink water after an hour or so.

Detoxification

"The "pollution" of our mind and body limits us from realizing our true potential. Time to time detox of your body and mind is key to explore the unlimited possibilities within you."

Every day we are exposed to pollutants, chemicals, metals, and pesticides. Our body detoxifies itself to some extent, but organs are burdened when there is a toxic overload. Hence they do not function properly. The liver gets sluggish, and toxins remain in our system. Because of this toxic overload, our body gives signs of tiredness, gas, bloating, pains, low energy, headaches, allergies, mental confusion, food cravings, bad breath, etc.

We are in constant contact with harmful organisms. Chemical toxins are ubiquitous in our environment.

Causes of accumulation of toxins in the body

- **Food:** Food is the biggest culprit in making our bodies toxic. Knowingly or unknowingly, we are consuming pesticides along with our food. Processed foods also add a lot of toxic load to our system. In the sugar refining process, Sulphur is being used to remove the impurities. As a result, Sulphur is retained in sugar and can cause harmful effects over some time. [28]

- **Water:** Sometimes tap water contains chlorine, fluoride, arsenic, lead, etc. [29]
- **Air:** Outside the house, one is exposed to polluted air, and inside the house, the use of chemicals, bleach, chemical-laden cosmetic products is rampant. [30]
- **Heavy metals:** Mercury is widely present in water resources such as rivers, lakes, and oceans. Excessive intake of fish may cause mercury toxicity. Mercury is often used in dental procedures like fillings in teeth. Cooking food in aluminum cookware causes the aluminum to accumulate inside the body. Protein supplements can be high in arsenic, lead, cadmium, and BPA. [31] Many protein powders have been tested, and most of them carry metals. These metals are required for the human body in small amounts, but they can become dangerous if taken in excess. Heavy metal toxicity can damage the brain, lungs, kidneys, and other organs. [32]
- **Usage of plastics:** Plastic enters our system when hot foods/ drinks are stored in plastic containers. BPA plastic bottles are much in usage, which is harmful to the body. [33]
- Personal care products like makeup, cosmetics, antiperspirants, etc., are also full of chemicals. [34]
- People who work in industries and mines are more prone to toxins. [35]

Detoxification means the removal of toxins from the body. It is cleansing and nourishing the body. Detoxification helps to deal with toxic overload.

There are different types of detoxifying diets. It is recommended to detox for 7 days or 14 days by consuming raw fruits and vegetables with nuts and seeds. Hydration in the form of plain water and warm water should be taken all day. Turmeric tea helps a lot during this process. Detox diet differs from person to person depending on individual needs and one's body type. Detox tea, as per Doshas, helps a lot in flushing out toxins. During the detox period, one should avoid sugar, caffeine, saturated fats, alcohol, meat, GMO food and switch over to natural raw foods. Consumption of fruits and vegetables helps our body to get rid of "ama." Detox diets are often high in fiber. During detox, one should not come in contact with chemical-based household cleaners, cosmetic products, and personal products.

The difference between fasting and detoxification is that fasting involves completely refraining from solid food for a certain period, and detoxification involves a higher intake of healthy and raw food. Detox can be done any time of the year but is more beneficial during spring. Proper sleep, yoga, deep breathing techniques, meditation, dry skin brushing, and massage facilitate the detox process. It is recommended to avoid intense and long workouts during detox. Plenty of rest, walk, yoga, and stretching are also beneficial. Detox diets have resulted in people feeling very light, more energetic, glow in the skin, and a reduction in body weight. It is a way to recharge and rejuvenate your body.

Tips to reduce or eliminate toxins

- Drink plenty of water to help the body to remove toxins through urine and sweat. One can have plain water, lemon water, or fruit-infused water. Water cleanses the body. Instead of using RO go for natural methods or basic water filters to purify the water. In winter, it is good to use copper vessels to store water, and during summer, earthenware is beneficial to store water.

- Practice nasal breathing instead of mouth breathing. Nasal breathing filters the air we breathe in. Use a breathing mask outdoors to get clean and filtered air. Nasal breathing while running provides more oxygen in the body cells and lowers the heart rate. Inhaling and exhaling from the nose is highly aerobic. [36]

- Use organic produce as much as possible. If organic produce is unavailable, wash the fruits and vegetables under tap water and soak them in a container with water and 1 tsp baking soda. Soak it for 15 minutes and rinse it again with plain water. By doing so, most of the pesticides get eliminated.

- Have probiotic-rich foods regularly.

- Avoid sugar and processed foods.

- Oil pulling is a great way to get rid of toxins from the oral cavity. On an empty stomach, take coconut oil in the mouth and swish all the sides. Do not swallow the oil. Keep it in the mouth for 15-20 minutes. Spit the oil and rinse the mouth with lukewarm water.

- Eat plenty of fiber-rich foods. Eat more fruits and vegetables.

- Reduce stress by practicing yoga and meditation.

- Avoid MSG (Monosodium glutamate) and ASPARTAME completely.

- Avoid plastic bottles and containers. Use steel, glass, or copper bottles.

- Ayurvedic massage helps detoxify the body. Massage boosts oxytocin hormone, which decreases anxiety and depression and boosts immunity. It improves lymphatic circulation as well as blood circulation. Massage helps in flushing out the toxins and wastes from the body.

- Sauna- Sauna or steaming is great heat therapy to dissolves toxins and lets you sweat them out.

- Nasya (nasal oiling)- Lubrication of the nasal passages with oil is called Nasya. Sesame oil, ghee, almond oil, mustard oil, and herbal oils can be used depending upon the type of Doshas. [37]

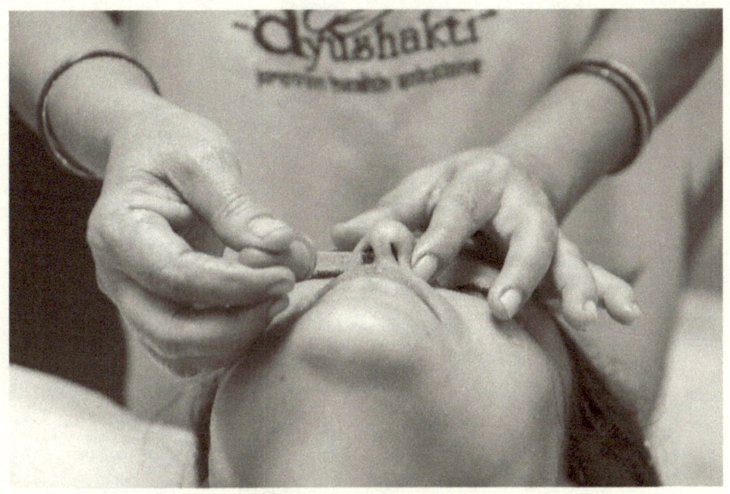

Picture 9: Nasya

It is one of the treatments used during the panchakarma process. Nasya keeps the mucosal lining lubricated and strong and prevents allergies and infections.

Liver Detoxification

The liver is one of the hardest working organs in our body. It detoxifies the blood, produces bile, removes toxins and excess estrogen from the body. It also stores many vitamins and minerals. To maintain the liver's optimal functioning, it is essential to detoxify it from time to time. The liver can be detoxified any time of the year; however, spring is the best season. Summer heat is hard on the liver, so it is better to detox the liver before summer.

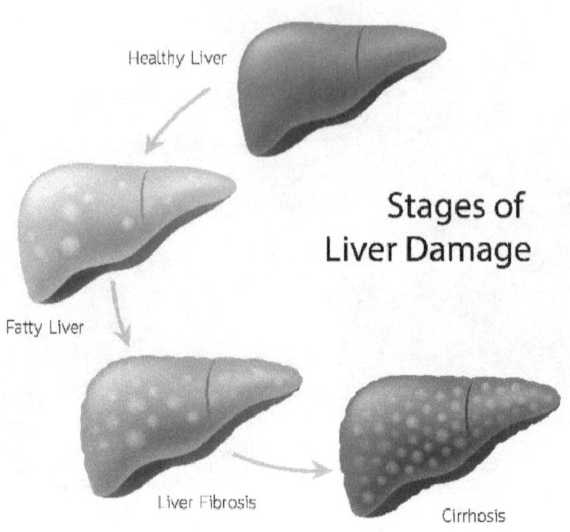

Picture 10: Stages of Liver damage

- Avoid all the Pitta aggravating drinks like tea, coffee, and alcohol.
- Have Kanji more often. (refer to probiotics chapter)
- Say YES to organic fresh fruits and vegetables.
- Say NO to processed foods like white flour products, unhealthy fats, and sugars.
- Have carrots, beets, and ginger juice to cleanse the liver.
- Eat a pitta pacifying diet. (refer to chapter "Ayurveda")
- Bhumi amla, Daruhaldi, Bhringraj, Kutki helps in cleansing and strengthening the liver.

Health benefits of detoxification

Boost energy: If you feel tired and lethargic all the time, it means it is time to detox.

Cleanses the liver: Pollutants, heavy metals, over usage of medications cause liver exhaustion. Non-alcoholic fatty liver is a common problem most of us face, and detoxification is a great way to eliminate the liver's fat molecules. After the detoxification, the liver functions much better.

Reduces inflammation: Eat more raw foods and healthy fats to help the body to eliminate inflammation.

Balances body's pH: [38] As we start eating raw fruits and veggies, which are alkaline, we can balance the pH and avoid most of the diseases since an acidic body is the hub of most serious diseases.

Healthy and clearer skin: Your skin reflects what you eat. By eating unhealthy processed foods, the skin produces acne, pimples, and blemishes. Detox reduces skin problems and gives a glow to the skin.

Aid weight loss: If you want to lose weight, detox is the best option as it increases metabolism and burns fat quickly.

Stronger immune system: People who fall sick easily and catch a cold and flu can increase their immunity by following a detox.

Better digestion and metabolism: The process of detox ensures that the body is not burdened with bad fat and sugar. As the athlete gets into natural eating, toxins are eliminated from the body. Drinking some detox drinks aids digestion, and the body absorbs nutrients optimally. It also maintains regular bowel movements.

Improve mental wellness: Detox aids in enhanced mental clarity. There is a significant decrease in the mental fog, and the mind opts to choose healthier foods.

Detoxing the body helps to get rid of unhealthy eating habits. Towards the end of the detox week, the body feels much lighter and happier. After detox, one can continue eating healthy food. During detox, the body still needs to consume nutrients to survive, so detoxification doesn't mean stop eating. It means choosing the right food at the right time and replacing bad food with healthy options.

For athletes, it's better to detox once or twice a year so that their body feels lighter and can achieve optimal performance in run events. Do not go for detoxifying diet just before the running event. 2-3 days after the main run, detoxification for 7 or 14 days is recommended.[39]

Fasting (Upvasa)

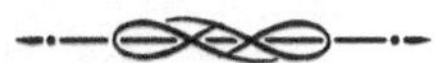

"If you want to be Fast in decision making, in athletic endeavors, in everything you do, then Fasting is a process you need to master."

Fasting means abstaining from all solid foods or eliminate a particular group of food from your diet for some time. The word "Fasting" is derived from 'feastan' which means to fast, observe and be strict. Fasting is usually done for religious purposes or health reasons. Fasting is a way to rest the digestive system. It has been practiced for thousands of years. When the body does not get food for longer periods, it starts to burn off glucose and fat. The body begins to form ketones, and this state is called ketosis.

In Ayurveda [40] one should undertake fasting as per their Doshas. Vata people should not fast for a long period. Doing so will aggravate more Vata in their body, which may damage the organs. They should take milk, honey, lemon, fruit juices, or warm herbal teas during the fasting period. Pitta people can fast on raw fruits and veggies. Kapha people can undertake regular fasting and should consume ginger tea. In Ayurveda, fasting is considered therapy to cure various health ailments. Overeating leads to an accumulation of waste and poisonous matter called "Ama." Digestion and elimination become slow. Fasting gives rest to the digestive system and re-ignites the digestive fire. The digestion of food and utilization of the nutrients is greatly improved after fasting. Fasting is the process of purification and an effective and quick method to cure various diseases.

Hippocrates, the father of modern medicine, states fasting is a path to rejuvenate the body, and it improves self-healing properties.

Types of Fasting

- 16/8 Intermittent fasting
- 24hrs protocol fasting
- Alternate day fasting
- Extended fasting
- Dry or No water fasting

Intermittent fasting: [41] This is an easy way of fasting. The most popular one is called the 16/8 time period, where one fast for 16 hours and the eating window is open for 8 hours. This is also called time-restricted eating. Eating two meals a day with one snack is the practice. It involves skipping one meal of the day. One can achieve 16 hours fast by having an early dinner and opting for a late breakfast the following day. During the fasting time, drink only water, green tea, and black coffee. Do not count calories; eat two nutritious, wholesome, healthy meals. If it is impossible to do it every day, one can also opt for weekdays only or thrice a week.

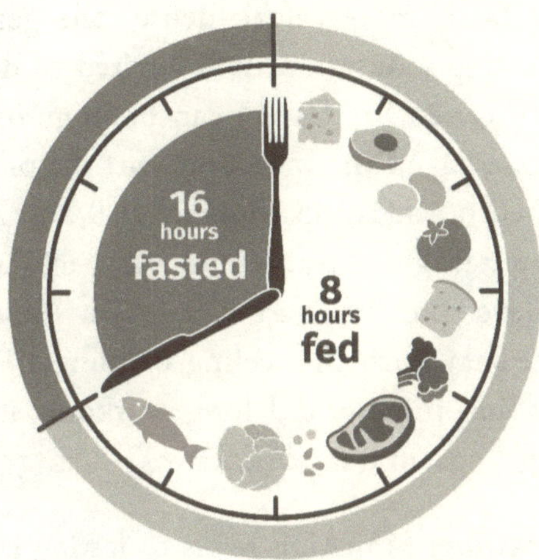

Picture 11: Intermittent fasting

Pick the 8-hour eating window period that best fits your routine. 16/8 intermittent fasting is a sustainable and easy way to fast for a healthy lifestyle.

Benefits

- Losing fat while maintaining muscle mass
- Weight loss
- Supports longevity
- Improves gut health
- Reduce inflammation
- Increases energy
- Improve immune system

24 Hours fasting: [42] means no food intake for 24 hours. One can plan to begin the fast from the dawn of a day till the dawn of the next day. E.g., If you had your breakfast at 9 am, then fast for 24hrs would mean eating the next day at 9 am. The meal consumed before fasting should be healthy and must include healthy fat. As fat is more calorie-dense, one gets a feeling of being full for a longer duration. It is advised to drink plenty of water while fasting. 24 hrs fasting can be done once or twice a week. Choose one day of the week and start the protocol. Let say you have finished breakfast on Monday at 9 am, and you begin fasting. Drink water, green tea, lemon water all day on Monday and Tuesday. Have your breakfast at 9 am on Tuesday. Green tea or Green coffee may curb the feeling of hunger. While fasting, abstain from doing intense and long workouts instead, opt to include walking, yoga, and meditation.

Alternate-day fasting: [43] ADF refers to fasting every other day. On fasting days, one can drink water, lemon water, green tea, black tea, green coffee, and black coffee. In case of hunger pangs, fruits can be had. This way of fasting is very effective for weight loss. People who are at the borderline for diabetes can lose weight and can manage their blood sugar levels by ADF.

Extended fasting: [44] Extended fasting is abstaining from eating for more than 48 hours and can last up to a week. This fasting is usually undertaken by people who have experience with other types of fasting. This is more advanced fasting [45]. It is the most ancient and powerful strategy for healing. It activates maximum autophagy, which means the body eats up damaged cells, and then there is the creation of new cells.

Dry or No Water fast: [46] In this type of fasting, people don't eat or drink anything. This is also called "Nirjala" fast. Nirjala means fasting without the intake of water. This is extremely beneficial for cell repair. Like extended fasting, this is also an advanced fasting method. Usually, a dry fast is advisable for not more than 24 hours.

Benefits of all kinds of fasting

- Lightness in the body
- Weight loss
- More energy
- Increases the secretion of growth hormone
- Reduces total cholesterol levels
- Improves digestion
- Increases longevity
- Improves brain function
- Improves Immune system
- Fights premature aging
- Increases autophagy

Fasting can be challenging for many, but one must find an easy way of doing it. Always start by making minor changes in the eating patterns and timings and gradually increase the fasting timings. During fasting days, light yoga, walk, and stretches can be done. Fasting makes the person strong. Many diseases have their origin in overeating, so through fasting, one can cure many diseases. Practicing fasting does not mean that you can eat junk food during the non-fasting period. The full benefit of fasting can be achieved by staying away from processed foods and drinking plenty of water on fasting days.

Breaking fast is also an important aspect. When the fast is completed, abstain from consuming heavy foods immediately. Intake of fruits, dates, dry fruits, nuts, khichdi on the first two days post-fast is recommended. After that, one can gradually start incorporating other food items. If the transition to eating solid foods is carefully planned, there won't be any discomfort. During the transition period, rest well, do not go for intense workouts.

Fasting is not recommended for elite marathoners; however, recreational athletes can fast during their recovery phase of training.

During the recovery phase, you can follow a 24hours or more fasting protocol. Instead of doing the regular workouts, go for a walk and yoga. Moreover, if you want to do it in everyday life, then intermittent fasting for 12-15 hours should be fine for recreational athletes. A pre-workout meal is essential for endurance sports.

Simple steps for beginners

- The first step is to find out the reason to fast. Understand whether it is for a spiritual purpose, weight loss, to maintain the fitness levels, or is it to address some health issues.
- Once a person decides to fast, it is advisable to start fasting for a short duration and gradually increase the timings.
- Stay hydrated with water and other fluids.
- Keep a variety of fruits and veggies at home.
- Do not store unhealthy processed food at home.
- Listen to one's body and make changes accordingly.

Precautions Before beginning to fast, consult a doctor and follow the process under medical supervision, especially if one is on medications that need to be taken with food.

Women who are trying to conceive, pregnant, and breastfeeding mothers should not follow fasting. If you are in a growing stage, underweight, malnourished, anorexia, or suffering from severe illness, refrain from fasting.

Finally, when fasting, listen to your body. It shouldn't be extremely uncomfortable. Minor discomfort is normal; however, if it's getting awful, then better to break the fast and have some light food.

Note: Please consult your family physician before following any fasting protocol.

Nutrition for Athletes

*"Personal Bests happens when
three things fall in place: Rest-Work-Recovery.
Nature provides you a solution for all three."*

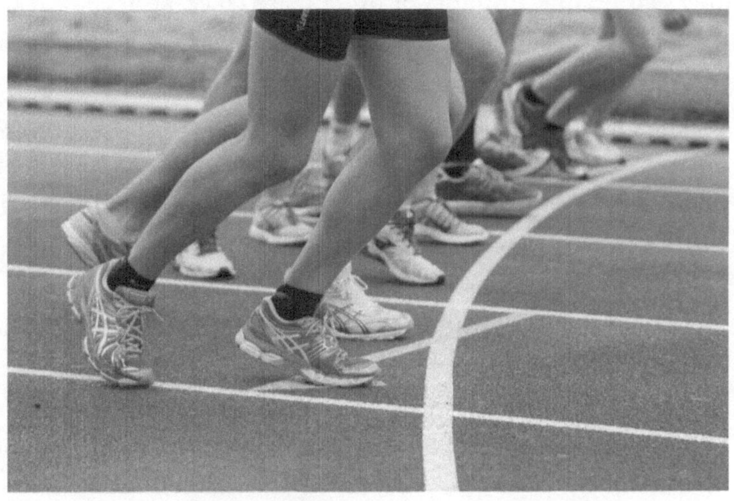

Picture 12: Athletes

Who is an Athlete?

An athlete is a person who competes in sports that involve physical strength, speed, or endurance. Athletes may be amateurs or professionals.

What is Nutrition?

Nutrition is the process of obtaining food for health and for physical and mental growth. The word nutrition first appeared in 1551 and came from the Latin word nutritive means "to nourish." It's about eating a healthy and balanced diet. The food we eat contains nutrients. Nutrients are substances required to perform various functions in the body. Proper nutrition is one of the most important factors to realize full athletic potential. In the current food industry, athletes take a very high carb diet/isolated proteins/Keto diet. Keto diets are good only for a short period, but in the long term, it deprives the athlete of other healthy nutrients. Too much protein is also not good for kidneys. The body can absorb only a small portion of protein at a time, and if large amounts of protein are taken at one go, it does not get absorbed and may lead to kidney disease or deposit in the form of uric acid on the joints. It is better to take different sources of food in divided dosage to get the right nutrition. A balanced breakfast is better than replacing them with protein supplements. Though eggs are a wholesome diet in itself, combining them with other fibrous foods increases their absorption value. It is important to eat low glycemic carbs. If one wants a lean muscular physique, along with protein, it is essential to include carbs as well. No or low carb diet can lead to muscle catabolism if one works in a fasted state or for a longer duration at high intensities. Rather than dividing the food into these categories, we should eat a balanced and wholesome meal.

Glycemic index: Glycemic index (GI) gives us an idea about how our body converts carbohydrates into glucose. It simply measures how quickly a food causes blood sugar levels to spike. Foods with high GI cause a rapid rise in blood sugar. However, foods with low GI absorb slowly, and there is a slower rise in blood sugar. Low glycemic index foods can help to lose body fat and increase lean muscle mass. It also improves energy levels in endurance athletes.

Low GI carbs digest slowly to provide a steady supply of blood sugar; that's why the emphasis is given to low to medium GI carbs during event runs. The glycemic index values range from 0-100. Low GI food means less than 55. Low and medium GI foods should be incorporated.[47]

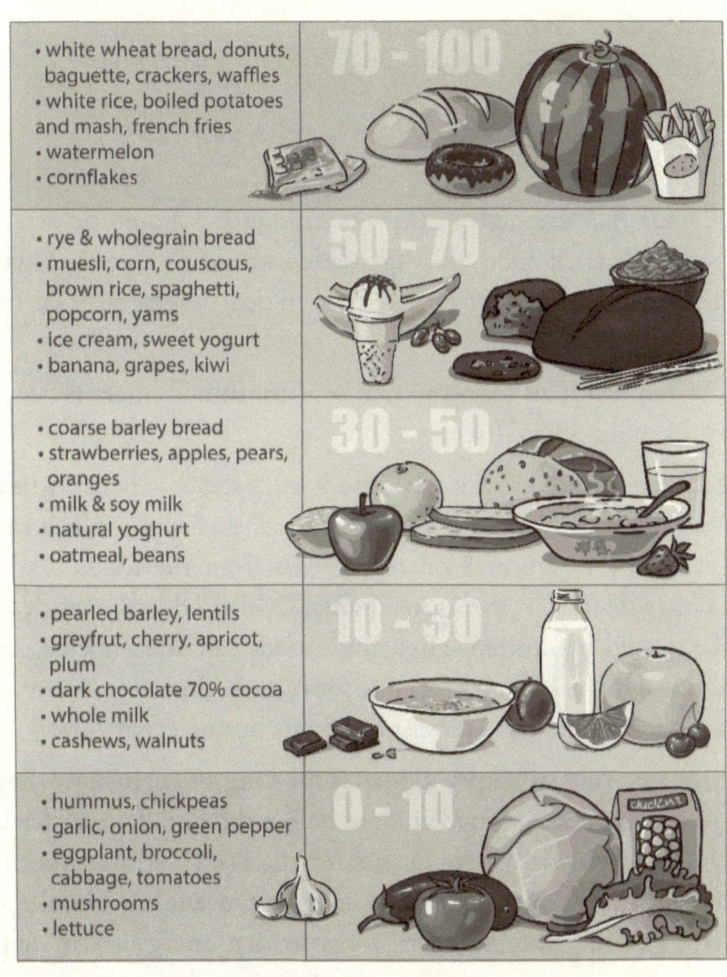

Picture 13: Glycemic Index

List of low glycemic foods good for athletes

- Rolled Oats
- Whole wheat
- Buckwheat (kuttu)
- Ragi
- Peanuts
- Vegetables like Cauliflower, tomatoes, green beans, carrots, bottle gourd, sweet potatoes, leafy greens
- All types of Lentils and legumes
- Milk, curd, paneer, cheese
- Nuts
- Seeds

Foods that are high in the glycemic index should be avoided. Examples of such food are sugar-laden breakfast cereals, biscuits, white bread, all kinds of desserts, sweetened beverages, fried food, etc.

When real food found in nature is consumed, there is no need to count calories or GI scores.

Athletes need to learn what foods are good for energy, when to eat, how to eat, and what to eat to replenish their activity. It is better to get all the macro and micronutrients from the foods that one eats rather than from the supplements. During athletic events, fiber intake should be limited. High fiber foods can affect the digestive system and make it uncomfortable for runners during their runs. It's always advisable to have fewer fiber foods during event runs.

Do not run an empty stomach for long or intense workouts. Some snacks would be good an hour before the run. Eating a healthy snack before exercise serves as fuel for the body and maximizes an athlete's efforts and results. It also helps to prevent low blood sugar. It helps in filing the glycogen stores so that energy levels remain elevated during workouts. Few days before and on the event day, concentrate more on carbohydrates because carbohydrates are easily converted to glucose than proteins and fats. The second most important function of carbohydrates is the protein-sparing property. This means if one does not consume an adequate amount of carbs before an event, then protein will provide the energy and not preserve muscles. So, it's important to include low GI carbs food.

Some nutrition guidelines for athletes, which they can regularly follow to achieve their goals are-

- Start your day with room temperature or warm water depending upon the weather and Prakriti of a person. Never drink cold water.
- Always have fruits empty stomach.
- Hydrate well, but do not drink water along with your meals as this disrupts digestion.
- Lunch should be the biggest meal of the day. It should be wholesome, including all the food groups. Must include curd or buttermilk for lunch.
- Dinner should be early and light consisting of easily digestible vegetables. Eat dinner 3-4 hours before bedtime.
- Have sound sleep

Pre-workout food is a snack or a meal taken 1-3 hours before the workout. A pre-workout meal is essential to prevent muscle glycogen depletion during workouts and also reduces muscle protein breakdown.

One size doesn't fit all. The same rule applies here. One food doesn't work for all. Try different foods during your training runs and see what works best for you.

Pre-Workout food options

- Raw banana powder porridge

- Sweet potato/Potato and nut butter
- Banana and nut butter
- Curd, banana, and honey
- Rolled oats porridge
- Cooked Beetroot juice and unsalted nuts
- Raw organic honey sandwich
- Peanut butter and sandwich
- Bulletproof coffee

Carbohydrates are the main key food for athletes. Along with carbs, essential amino acids and some fat are also important.

Each individual is unique. Everyone has a different digestion time. Pre-workout food can be had 60 minutes before running. If the feeling of fullness is there, then move the pre-workout meal timings to 90 minutes before the run. Listening to one's body and moving the timings forward or backward is essential.

To avoid "hitting the wall," endurance athletes load up on carbs a few days before an event. In this way, they can maximize the storage of glycogen in the liver and muscles. Simple carbohydrates give a short-term energy boost. After a while, athletes may feel a drop in energy. Complex carbohydrates provide energy more consistently. They are hitting the wall or bonking means that the muscles have used up all the stored glycogen and are then dependent on other nutrients to support energy levels. It's run out of energy. The first primary source of energy is glycogen, and the second is fat—the greater the body's ability to store glycogen, the greater the ability to perform well. If you hit the wall, then slow down and eat or drink carbs regularly in intervals. It is not advisable for an easy or short run to have large carb meals because the body will end up storing fats due to excess carbs that are not getting burnt at all. With proper training and a diet plan, one can easily overcome bonking.

Tip to maximize your glycogen stores

Glycogen stores can be maximized or maintained by eating carbohydrates rich diet. Most of the athletes pay attention only to protein. One should have carbs rich diet a few days before an event with essential amino acids and some fat for good glycogen stores.

What foods to avoid in pre-workout nutrition

- Fried food – Results in sluggish digestion.
- Milk products – Results in gastrointestinal issues.
- Heavy meals – Avoid large, heavy meals before your workout/ race.
- High Sugary and processed food – Gives instant energy but can result in gastrointestinal (GI) issues.

Intra-run nutrition

For longer runs, fueling at regular intervals is important. When one runs for more than 90 minutes, the muscle glycogen is depleted, and soon, the body runs out of energy. It depends upon how many glycogen stores one has. It usually depletes anywhere between 90 to 120 minutes. Hydrate well with electrolytes, as discussed in the next chapter. Every 45-60 minutes of the run, have banana/orange (Chew orange and throw the fiber)/soft dates/raisins/honey or jam sandwich/homemade energy bars.

It's recommended that one should fuel their body with the right amount of nutrients. [48]

Nutrient	Daily Requirement	Pre-Exercise	During Exercise	Post-Exercise
Carbohydrate	6-10 g/kg/day (1-3 h/day)	2 gm/kg 1hr prior workout. 3 gm/kg 2hrs prior workout. 4 gm/kg 3hrs prior workout	60–70 g/h (>2.5 h)	1.0–1.2 g/kg/h (first 3–5 h)
Protein	~0.3 g/kg every 3–5 h throughout the day	0.3 g/kg	5 g/h (BCAA or EAA)[49]	0.3 g/kg within 0–2 h
Fat	Do not restrict to <20% total caloric energy.	Avoid	Avoid	Omega 3, DHA supplements to help recovery
Hydration	Follow thirst mechanism, monitor parameters (body weight, urine color)	2hr prior have 10ml/kg body weight	~400–800 mL/h Do a sweat test for specificity	10ml/kg body weight per hour for the next two hours.
Sodium	300–600 mg/h if high sweat rate. Adjust intake according to individual athlete variations based on sweat test.			
Nitrates	300–600 mg of nitrate (up to 10 mg/kg or 0.1 mmol/kg) or 500 mL beetroot juice or 3–6 whole beetroots within 90 min of exercise onset			
Caffeine	3–6 mg/kg taken 30–90 min before exercise			

Table 2

Post-Workout food

It should be a combination of carbohydrates and protein in the ratio of 4:1. Post-workout nutrition minimizes muscle breakdown and helps in the rebuilding process.

Post-Workout food options

- Paneer wheat wrap/sandwich and fresh juice (apple/orange/ pineapple)
- Curd rice
- Peanuts Poha (Rice flakes) and Buttermilk
- Ragi malt
- Peanut butter sandwich and Banana
- Fresh fruit juice and egg sandwich
- Hummus and pita bread
- Coconut water and kidney beans rice/wrap
- Homemade nuts and oats energy bars with milk
- Idli with peanut chutney
- Sprouts and potato salad
- Beet, apple, and nuts salad
- Sattu made with roasted gram flour. This composition is one of the highest sources of vegetarian protein and quality that is most easily absorbed by the body. 60 grams (4 tbsp) of this roasted flour gives 19.7 grams of high-quality protein along with Calcium and Magnesium

Sattu Porridge

Prep: 10 mins Cook: 5-7 mins;

Ingredients

- 2 Tablespoons sattu mix

- 1 cup water
- 1 cup milk
- 2 Tablespoons Sugar/Jaggery/Dates puree

Method

- Dissolve sattu mix in some water. Add milk
- Cook on low flame, stirring continuously to avoid lump formation.
- Add sugar/jaggery/dates puree as per taste.
- You can adjust the quantity of water/milk, depending on how thick you want.

Eating a healthy snack/meal after a workout builds muscle, aids fast recovery, and burns more fat. The right diet will help in quick recovery. Post-workout meal replenishes glycogen stores and initiates protein synthesis.

Sweet Potatoes are rich in Vitamins A and C. It is a good source of beta-carotene, manganese, and copper. Sweet potatoes are rich in carbohydrates hence is the best fuel for athletes.

Sweet potatoes can be boiled and baked. It's a perfect fueling food during long runs. It can be had as it is or mixed with other ingredients.

Sweet Potato and Nuts

Prep: 10 mins Cook: Nil;

Ingredients

- 1-2 boiled/baked sweet potato
- 2 walnuts

- 5 almonds
- Two teaspoons raw organic honey
- ¼ teaspoon Himalayan pink salt/sea salt

Method

- Chop the cooked sweet potatoes.
- Cut the nuts into small pieces.
- Mix them with honey and salt.
- The sweet potato and nuts mix are ready to eat.

Potatoes are an excellent source of potassium which is essential for muscles. It's easily digestible and provides both physical and mental strength.

Potatoes can be baked, boiled, and sautéed. Stay away from fried potatoes.

Rolled Oats is a good pre-run meal. It is easy to digest and provides a steady stream of energy. Go for rolled or steel-cut oats over instant.

Boil oats in water/milk, then add honey and 1 tsp of chopped nuts.

Beetroot contains nitrates, which convert into nitric oxide inside the body. Nitric oxide has several health benefits for athletes. It improves stamina, speed, and endurance.

Beetroot helps keep the blood pressure low, improves blood flow, and provides more oxygen to working muscles. Oxygen-rich blood helps one to workout longer and harder. It enhances aerobic performance. To ensure there are no digestive issues after having beetroot juice, one can steam the beetroot first and then juice it.

Organic Raw Honey is a natural sweetener and easily absorbed in the body. Honey is made up of glucose and fructose. It's a good fuel food for longer runs. It can keep one running for longer.

Take as it is or dilute it in water. It can be added in oatmeals, or one can make honey sandwiches. It can be taken as a hydration mix during runs. It gives constant energy and improves muscle function, and acts as an anti-inflammatory.

Bananas make a good snack for runners before, during, and after the run. While sweating, we lose sodium and potassium, which results in muscle cramps. These lost minerals should be replaced. One medium banana has about 400 mg of potassium.

Banana is also rich in Vitamin B6 and antioxidants and is an energy booster. It's easy to carry a snack. Simply peel and eat.

Raw Banana Powder is packed with carbohydrates, vitamins, and minerals.

It is a source of energy required for athletes.

Raw Banana Porridge

Prep: 15 mins Cook: 10;

Ingredients

- 1 ½ tablespoon Raw Banana powder
- 150ml Water or Milk
- Organic Jaggery powder or Raw organic honey
- Pinch of Himalayan pink salt
- Optional- Nuts like cashew, walnuts, almonds, etc

Method

- Dissolve raw banana powder into room temperature water or milk until there are no lumps.

- Cook it over medium flame until it boils and thickens to a porridge consistency.
- You can add nuts if you want to make it richer.
- Add Jaggery or honey as per your taste.

You can use this as fuel too on the bike by adding more hot water to reduce the thickness.

Mix it in hot water and have it in as pre-workout nutrition.

Coffee impacts athletic performance. It gives instant energy, but after some time, the athlete crashes easily. That's where bulletproof coffee comes in to picture. Because the MCT oil and ghee help the coffee slowly release over time, it gives the athlete long-lasting energy. It gives satiety for longer hours.

Bulletproof Coffee

Prep: 10 mins Cook: 5;

Ingredients

- 1 teaspoon Coffee
- 1 ½ tablespoon Virgin coconut oil
- 1-2 tablespoon Ghee
- 90-100ml of full-fat coconut milk
- Optional- Raw organic honey

Method

- Make regular black coffee.
- Add coconut milk as per taste. If you like it black, you can skip adding coconut milk.

- Add coconut oil and ghee to the coffee.
- Add honey if required.

Use of cold-pressed organic coconut oil and organic grass-fed cow ghee is recommended. For beginners, start with a lower dose of oil and ghee and gradually increase the quantity. Start with half the amount mentioned above and gradually increase after few days. If you have an upset stomach/acidity, refrain from taking and start after few days with small quantity.

Khichdi and dal chawal (dal rice) works as a perfect meal one day before the run event. Also, it is best to completely avoid sugary and fried foods a day before the race day.

What to avoid during race days?

- Do not try new food items on the event day. You never know how the body reacts. Race day is not a good time to experiment with anything new.
- For breakfast, avoid sugary cereals. Too much sugar gives the false energy spike.
- Fatty foods should be avoided as it takes longer time to digest.
- Though a high fiber diet is good on a regular day, it is not recommended on race day. It can upset the stomach.
- Increase the complex carbohydrates on race day but don't overdo.
- Have a light, complex carb dinner the day before an event. Do not have a large dinner.
- Shun alcoholic beverages 48 hours before the race.
- Avoid NSAIDs on a race day.

Hydration

*"For long, "Water" was the only drink we required
to quench our thirst and re-energize ourselves;
it had all the required minerals to keep us
healthy till we started processing it too."*

Every cell, tissue, and organ in our body needs water to survive and to function properly. It's important to stay hydrated before, during, and after the workout. Water transports nutrients to every part of the body. It regulates the body temperature and allows muscles to contract properly. It also removes the waste and toxins from the body.

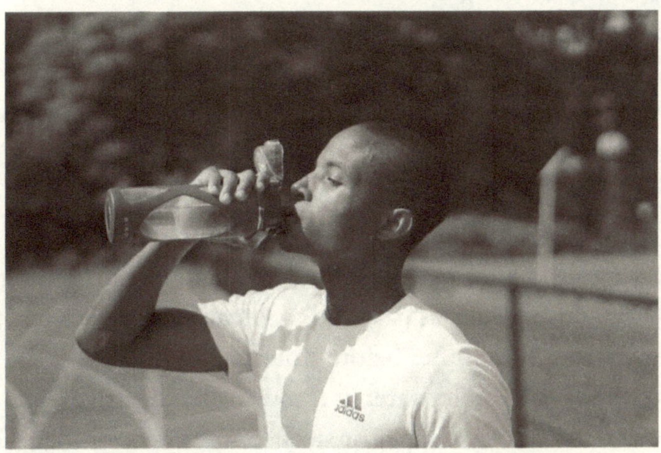

Picture 14: Athlete hydrating

A Dehydrated body does not give high performance. As athletes sweat a lot, they lose water and electrolytes. If they do not replenish, that could result in dizziness, muscle cramps, palpitations, nausea, and vomiting. Water loss depends on many factors like the intensity of the exercise, external temperature, humidity, and body weight. Muscle cramps can be because of low electrolytes in the body.

Electrolytes are responsible for maintaining the balance of fluids between the intracellular and extracellular environments, helps in muscle contractions, controlling PH balance. Electrolyte imbalance can cause a muscle spasm, fatigue, dizziness, constipation, nausea, dry skin, dry mouth, etc. There are several ways we can hydrate our bodies. For short workouts, water may be enough, but electrolytes should be added to water for long and intense workouts.

Athletes chug a big amount of water in one go, which does not get absorbed properly. Here are few tips on how to get good absorption of water.

Tips to effectively absorb water

- Sip water, do not gulp.
- Start mornings with lukewarm water.
- Have more water during day time than at night.
- Drink small sips of water frequently throughout the day. The body cannot absorb large volumes of water in a short duration of time.
- Do not have water along with meals. If too much water is taken with meals, digestion will be hindered, and one may suffer from digestive issues such as gas, acidity, bloating, stomachache, etc.
- Have water 30 minutes before a meal.
- Do not have ice-cold water as it lowers the digestive fire.
- Store water in clay/copper or steel containers or bottles. Do not store in plastic bottles.

Sports drinks are beverages that help athletes to rehydrate and replenish electrolytes. They are rich in water, sugar, and electrolytes. Many sports drinks contain electrolytes but also contain high amounts of sugar. They are more in calories, leading to weight gain and a risk factor for type 2 diabetes. High sugary sports drink also contribute to dental erosion.

Some liquids that pull hydration out of the body are caffeinated beverages, soda, and alcohol. These liquids cannot be considered as hydration drinks, so best to abstain from them.

Go for natural or homemade drinks instead of readymade sports drinks

- **Mix Water, lemon, honey, and sea salt**. This drink boosts hydration. You get the electrolytes from honey and salt without adding any chemicals. It also increases energy. It facilitates weight loss too. Regular intake reduces the inflammation from the body, prevents muscle cramps, and balances the body ph.
- **Buttermilk with Himalayan pink salt** provides minerals required by the body and helps to replenish the body's electrolyte levels.
- **Cow Milk** has a natural balance of nutrients. It has sodium and a large amount of potassium to restore the food balance after an exercise. It is a good recovery drink.
- **Coconut water** has a good amount of potassium and other nutrients, which help the body to hydrate. Mix pink salt or sea salt in coconut water.
- **Fruit juices** have 85% water content which makes them super hydrating. Do not opt for packaged fruit juices. Always have fresh juice with no sugar. Fruit juices are full of vitamins and minerals. Dilute it with equal quantities of water and add salt.

- **Green tea with honey-** Iced green tea with honey is great for improving endurance.

Hydration Mix

Prep: 5 mins

Ingredients

- 50gms of glucose
- 0.5gms of Himalayan pink salt
- 1.5grams of baking soda
- 500 ml of cold water
- one lemon or one orange

Method

- Juice either a lemon or orange and strain it.
- Mix it with cold water and add the rest of the ingredients.
- Your hydration mix is ready.

Research has been conducted on **pomegranate juice** and **kokum juice**. We can use equal quantities of pomegranate and kokum juice and also add cumin powder for gastric upset tummies during runs. This sports drink has anti-inflammatory properties as well. [50]

All hydration drinks must be sipped and not gulped to avoid gastric distension.

Avoid caffeinated beverages such as black tea, coffee, cola. These are not recommended for hydration. Caffeine is mildly diuretic. [51]

Pre-run hydration- A day before an event, drink more water. Two hours before the run, have 1-2 glasses of fluids. You can have fresh fruit juice diluted with equal quantities of water and 2 pinches of Himalayan pink salt. Another option is to have honey, lemon, and salt mixed with water. Thirty minutes before the event, drink a glass of water. Drink approximately 5–10 mL/kg body weight of hydration 2 hrs before exercise to ensure one is well hydrated before a workout that is longer than 2 hours [52]

Hydration during the run- for long runs, sip electrolyte water every 15-20 minutes in summer and every 25-30 minutes in winters. Drink according to thirst.

Post-run hydration- After finishing the run, drink homemade energy drinks. Hydration is extremely important after the run also.

Compare your weight before and after your long workout to find out your hydration needs. Weight loss of around 2% to 3% is acceptable. Above 3% may decrease subsequent endurance performance.

Energy drinks are classified into three categories-

Isotonic drinks- Isotonic drinks are similar to the human body's concentrations of electrolytes in the blood. It's ideal for endurance workouts. It contains 4 to 8 gm of sugar. If an athlete's workout lasts for more than an hour, it is important to have isotonic drinks. 1000ml of water, 200ml of any fruit squash, and half a teaspoon of salt make an isotonic solution.

Hypotonic drinks- They get absorbed very fast in the body but not for replenishing energy levels. It has a lower concentration of electrolytes than the human body. It contains 3 to 4 gm of sugar. These types of drinks are ideal for shorter and less intense workouts. 1000ml of water, 100ml of fruit squash, and ¼th teaspoon of salt make a hypotonic solution.

Hypertonic drinks- It's more concentrated than blood. It contains 8 or more than 8 gm of sugar. It's used for recovery after the exercise. 1000ml of water, 400ml of fruit squash, and half a teaspoon of salt make a hypertonic solution.

For proper hydration, it's important to understand one's personal hydration needs. How much fluid one needs to take depends upon several factors such as intensity and duration of workouts, temperature, humidity, and sweat rate.

Steps to check one's sweat rate

- Check weight before a workout
- Fluid intake during exercise
- Post-exercise body weight
- Workout duration
- Urine output

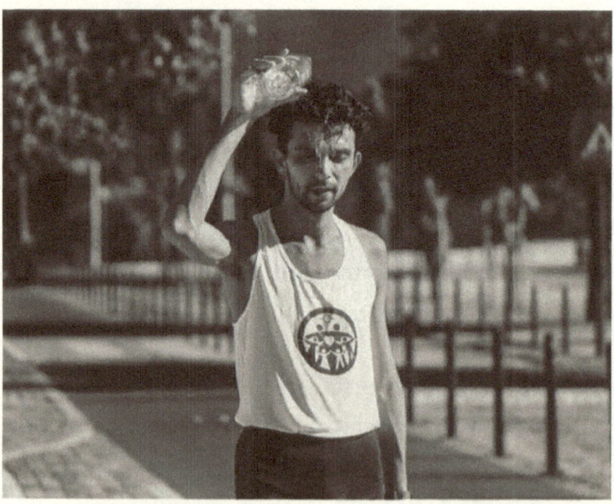

Picture 15: Athlete cooling his body

If there is a weight loss immediately after a workout, it means the athlete needs to hydrate more. If there is a gain in weight after a workout, then hydrate less. Sweat rate calculations data is generally recommended for less than 2 hours workout as after this period athletes burn glycogen during exercise which can give the wrong body weight.

Hyponatremia

Hyponatremia occurs when the sodium concentration in the blood gets abnormally low. This happens in athletes when they drink too much water. Athletes are aware of dehydration during marathons, so sometimes they over hydrate. When we over hydrate our body, sodium gets diluted, and cells swell up. This causes nausea, vomiting, bloating, muscle cramp, headache, confusion, and disorientation.

If one takes plain water for longer runs and does not consume sodium, they are prone to hyponatremia. Secondly, athletes who sweat a lot and don't take sodium during longer running events are also on the verge of hyponatremia.

Hyponatremia can be prevented if one is aware of fluid intake and the rate at which sweat is generated. So, include drinks with sodium and potassium in them and snack on salty foods during race days. Do not force drink water if the stomach is full.

Hypernatremia

Hypernatremia means too much sodium in the blood. It occurs when we take too much sodium or less intake of water. This causes excessive thirst, fatigue, muscle twitching, confusion. Hypernatremia can be prevented in athletes by replenishing fluids.

Hypo and hypernatremia are common electrolyte abnormalities that can be taken care of with proper hydration. Excess or deficit water is the main cause of these imbalances.

Muscle Cramps

Exercise-Associated Muscle Cramp (EAMC) is a sudden involuntary spasm that occurs in various muscles. This is a common problem in long-distance runners. The muscles of the calf or foot cramp easily during or after runs. Muscles become painful, hard, and sometimes swell.

Several factors can trigger cramps in muscles during long runs-

- Lactic acid builds up
- Neuromuscular hyperactivity [53]
- Not stretching enough before the run
- Dehydration
- Low sodium levels
- Poor blood circulation
- Magnesium/Potassium/Calcium deficiency
- Decreased oxygenation of the blood

Tips to prevent muscle cramps during runs-

- Hydrate well. Take electrolytes for long distances runs. (check "Table 2" in "Nutrition for athletes" chapter for recommended values)
- Regular massages make the muscles strong
- Take magnesium supplements
- Always stretch enough before and after runs
- Use compression socks during/after the run
- Use foam rollers post-run
- Apply Ice/heat- Apply ice first and then switch to warm post 48 hours of your workout.
- Include more strength training along with regular workouts

If you cramp during a run, do not force yourself to run further. Stop running, stretch, take deep breaths and start with a run/walk strategy.

DIY Solution for Leg Cramps

Cramp Solution

Prep: 10 mins

Ingredients

- 50ml of Apple Cider Vinegar
- 10ml Ginger Juice (without any fiber)
- 10ml Garlic Juice (without any fiber)

Method

- Juice a piece of fresh ginger and strain it.
- Juice 2-3 bulbs of garlic and strain it
- Mix them with vinegar, and your magic potion is ready to be carried during runs.

At the first sign of cramps, mix 10-15 ml with 25-30ml of water and have it. Don't swallow it. Swirl it inside the mouth for a while. This tangy flavor will reset the neuromuscular activity.

Amino Acids

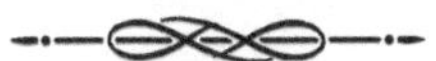

"Science has enabled us to be superior but it has also crippled us into being dependent on pharma even to stay healthy. There is a constant battle between Nature and Science. Science is winning. Hope it's the other way round soon."

Amino acids are the building blocks of proteins. They are organic compounds composed of nitrogen, carbon, oxygen, and hydrogen. Nitrogen is the addition of amino acids as compared to carbohydrates and fats. There are 20 different types of amino acids classified as essential and non-essential amino acids. The essential amino acid cannot be made on its own by the body. We need to take it from food sources. Non-essential amino acids are those that are produced by the body. Sources of essential amino acids are chicken, mutton, seafood, eggs, milk, and milk products. Lentils, legumes, nuts, seeds, millets are also good sources of amino acids. When we combine rice and lentils, it is a complete protein source. Khichdi, dal-chawal, rajma-chawal is considered a complete protein source. A complete protein is the one that provides all the essential amino acids.

Nine Essential Amino Acids

- Leucine
- Isoleucine
- Valine

These are considered as BCAA (explained in next topic)

- Phenylalanine
- Threonine
- Tryptophan
- Methionine
- Lysine
- Histidine

BCAAS's main function is muscle growth and repair. It eliminates fatigue, speeds up muscle growth, and lowers inflammation.

An anabolic state means that the body is building muscles.

A catabolic state means that the body is breaking down tissues. It refers to the breakdown of large molecules into smaller ones. Whenever we exercise, there is some tear/damage in our muscles.

If protein synthesis exceeds protein breakdown, one gains muscle, and if breakdown exceeds synthesis, then one loses muscle. Anabolism and catabolism are related to metabolism.

How to avoid the catabolic state

Catabolism can be avoided by training smart (including cardio as well as strength training), eating well, and taking adequate rest by sleeping for at least 7-8 hours. Intake of complex carbohydrates and proteins before, during and post-workout prevents catabolism. The body should be adequately nourished. Eat fruits, vegetables, nuts, seeds, whole grains, and good fats regularly.

BCAAs

Branched-chain amino acids are a group of three essential amino acids, which consist of leucine, isoleucine, and valine. These are called essential amino acids because our body cannot produce them, and we need to derive them from our diet. These amino acids are stored in the liver and skeletal muscles. Amino acids are the building blocks of protein. BCAAs have several functions in our body. It plays an important role in energy production, reduces fatigue during exercise, increases muscle mass, and enhances performance. People who face liver functioning issues can improve their health with an intake of BCAA. During long workouts, it's essential to take EAA (Essential Amino Acids) or BCAA.

Essential Amino Acids (EAA) rich foods

- Chicken breast
- Turkey
- Eggs
- Fish
- Dairy products like milk, curd, paneer, cheese
- Nuts- Almonds, Cashews, Walnuts
- Lentils
- Kidney Beans
- Chickpeas
- Whole wheat
- Roasted peanuts
- Moringa leaves

Glutamine

Glutamine is also an important amino acid for athletes. This is a non-essential amino acid that is synthesized by the body. This is beneficial to athletes who perform intense workouts. It is present in the lungs and skeletal muscles. When the athlete feels exhausted during runs due to a lactic acid build-up in muscles, glutamine delays muscle exhaustion. It also boosts immunity. [54]

Glutamine rich foods

- Seafood
- Eggs
- Paneer
- Chicken breast
- Mutton
- Milk
- Cabbage
- Kidney and black beans
- Sauerkraut

The egg is a wholesome diet in itself, and thereby, the entire egg, along with the yolk, should be consumed. Eggs are a great source of Omega 3 fatty acid which acts as an anti-inflammatory. It is rich in Vitamin A, D, and E. Unless restricted by a physician, do include egg yolks in moderation.

During regular days take nutrients from food, but during long training workouts or events, it is impossible to eat big meals, so intake of supplements is recommended.

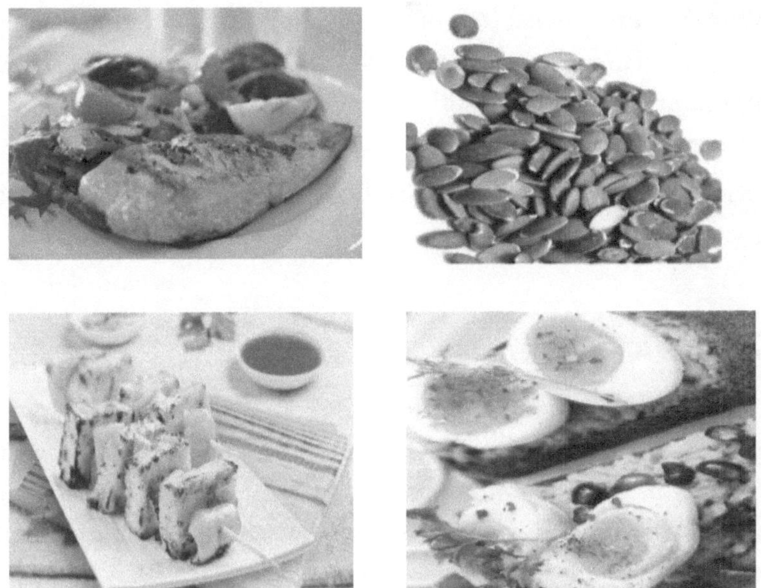

Picture 16: Food rich in Amino Acids

Non-Essential Amino Acids

Arginine is a non-essential amino acid that plays an important role for athletes. It directly increases the nitric oxide activity in the body. Food sources rich in arginine are chicken, pumpkin seeds, soy, dairy products, and lentils [55]

Glutathione is made up of three amino acids- glutamine, glycine, and cysteine. Glutathione or GSH is an antioxidant produced in cells. It treats and prevents many diseases. Glutathione act as a detoxifier. While running long-distance, runners build up lactic acid in the muscles, which causes pain. Glutathione act as an anti-inflammatory that helps in relieving the pain. Thus, it helps in workout recovery also. It increases energy. Levels of Glutathione can be depleted due to many factors such as aging, poor diet, pollution, stress, toxins, and a sedentary lifestyle. One study showed that 90 minutes of exercise led to a 60% reduction in glutathione, leading to muscle fatigue, pain, and poor athletic performance. So, it's important to include glutathione for longer runs. [56]

Glutathione-rich foods are bone broth, whey protein, turmeric, asparagus, okra, cauliflower, cabbage, mustard greens, spinach, broccoli, garlic, etc.

Collagen

Collagen is a structural protein found in the bones, tendons, ligaments, and skin. As we age, the body produces less collagen. Collagen promotes healthy joints, increases muscle mass, improves muscle recovery, and is hence an important nutrient for athletes. It helps to rebuild the connective tissues. The stronger the connective tissues, the lower the risk of injuries. It improves athletic performance. Collagen is an ideal pre, intra, and post-workout nutrition as it restores and repairs the muscles. Collagen improves gut health by regulating stomach acid secretion. It also repairs the stomach and intestinal linings. Collagen supports healthier skin. It helps the skin cells to renew and repair.

A study conducted at Penn State University saw a significant improvement in activity-related joint pain in athletes.[57]

Foods rich in collagen are Bone broth, chicken, gelatin, and egg yolk.

Vegetarians can have proline and glycine-rich foods like soybeans, spirulina, milk and milk products, pumpkin seeds, sesame seeds, cabbage, and leafy greens.

An easier way to get collagen is to take a collagen peptide supplement in which proteins are broken down into smaller pieces (hydrolyzed) for easier digestion and absorption. Vitamin C helps in collagen synthesis; hence one must include vitamin c rich foods while taking collagen supplements.

There are several types of collagen-

Type I is linked with the skin

Type II is linked with cartilage and joint health

Type III is linked with bones, connective tissues. It is also important for the health of skin, hair, and nail.

With its growing popularity, plenty of different collagen supplements are available. Look for types I, II, III collagen supplements as per one's health goals. For athletes, go for type II collagen supplements.

Herbs for Athletes

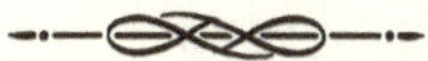

"When we have safer alternatives to performance-enhancing substances. Why not embrace it?"

The stress of performance is so high in many athletes that they start using enhancing drugs that are banned. These performance-enhancing substances (PES) come with severe side effects. PES causes high blood pressure, irregular heartbeat, headaches, muscle cramps, heart attack, stroke, thyroid problems, etc. This makes the need for safe and natural alternatives. Herbs are safe and natural options that provide endurance benefits. Here is the list of few herbs that athletes can use to enhance athletic performance.

- Ashwagandha
- Arjuna
- Triphala
- Moringa
- Turmeric
- Shatavari

Ashwagandha is also known as Indian Ginseng, the most powerful herb in Ayurveda. This herb act as an adaptogen which means it copes with one's body from stress. It promotes both physical and mental health. Ashwagandha decreases the hormone cortisol and increases testosterone. It reduces LDL cholesterol and triglycerides.

It improves cardiac health and overall well-being. This herb increases energy levels, reduces fatigue, and promotes muscle growth. Ashwagandha is a must for the better performance of athletes. Many studies were done about the effects of supplementation with ashwagandha on VO2max. Studies showed that it improved VO2max in athletes.[58]

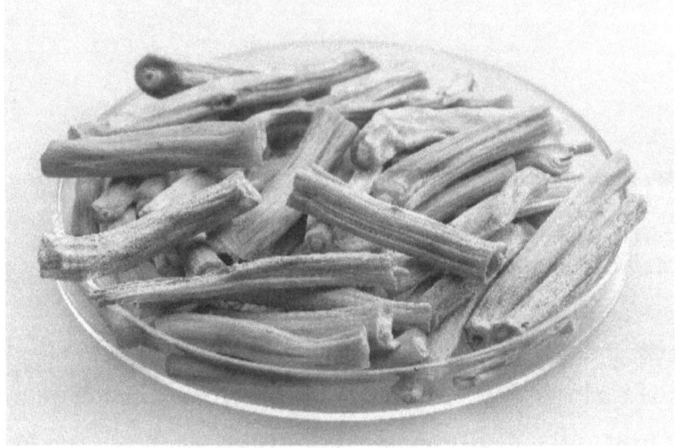

Picture 17: Ashwagandha

In Ayurveda, Ashwagandha is described as balya, which means it gives inner strength. The standard dosage of Ashwagandha is 500mg twice a day with water. 2 weeks before the event, this dosage can be increased.

Arjuna (Terminalia Arjuna) This herb is a powerful heart tonic. It's rich in COQ-10, which provides energy to the cells. Arjuna maintains healthy cholesterol levels and strengthens the heart muscle. It is considered as hrdya dravya in Ayurveda. [59]

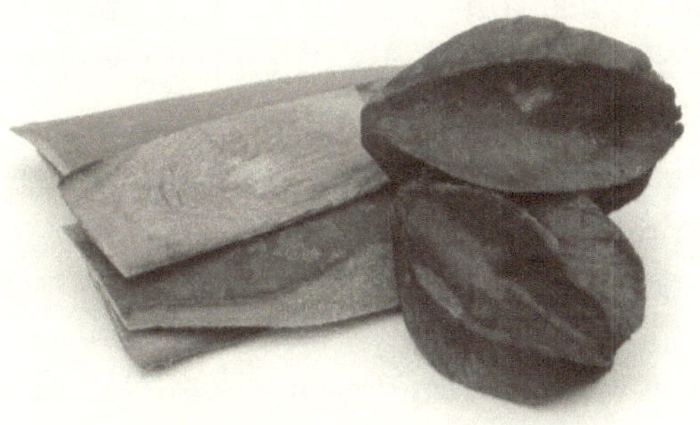

Picture 18: Arjuna Bark

For athletes, Ashwagandha and Arjuna in combination show great benefits. In combination, it has been seen that VO2 max and velocity are improved. Arjuna improves cardiac efficiency. It has cardioprotective and antihypertensive properties. It improves ejection fraction and reduces heart rate. The dosage of Arjuna is 500mg twice a day with water. This dosage can be increased 2 weeks before the event.

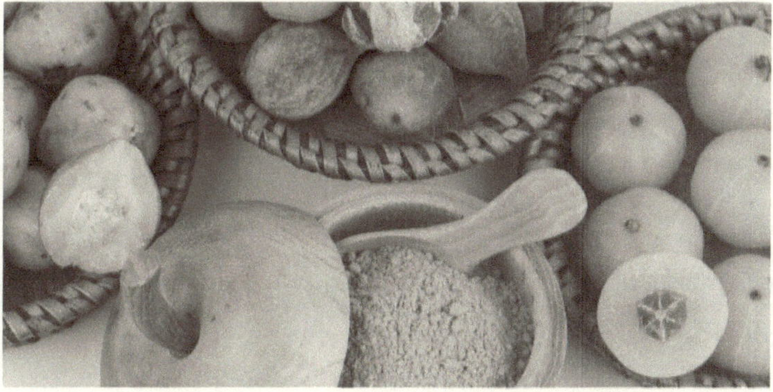

Picture 19: Triphala

Triphala is a combination of three fruits: Amla, Bibhitaki, and Haritki. Due to wrong eating habits, toxins build up in our system, which is called Ama. Triphala works on this Ama and helps to get rid of toxins from the digestive tract. Triphala balances all the Doshas. It helps in weight loss. It cleanses the colon and strengthens the intestine muscles. It can be taken at night or in the morning on an empty stomach with lukewarm water. For a dull and sluggish feeling, Triphala helps to detox the body and balance digestion. Triphala is available in powder, capsule, and tablet forms.[60]

Moringa is a superfood having amazing health benefits. It contains a variety of proteins, vitamins, minerals, and other nutrients. It has a good amount of calcium too.

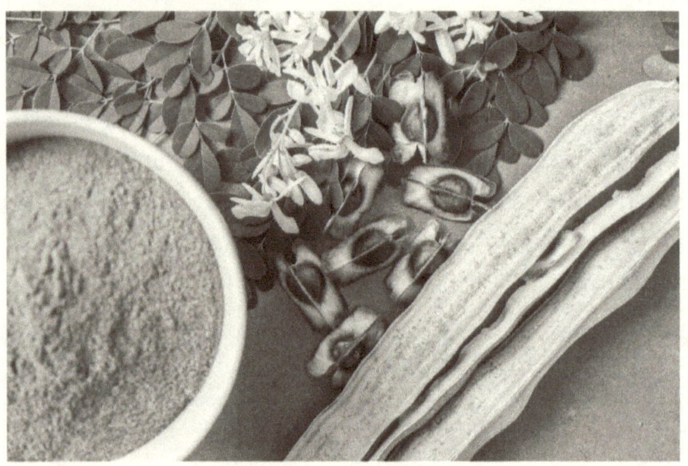

Picture 20: Moringa

Regular intake of moringa leaf powder can fulfill calcium's daily requirement, about 75% of iron and 50% of protein. It's a rich source of vitamins A and C. It acts as an anti-inflammatory and treats edema. It protects the cardiovascular system by reducing cholesterol and prevents plaque formation. Moringa is available in powder and capsule form. The powder can be mixed in water or soup, smoothies, juices, lentil curry, or any other food. [61]

Turmeric has curcumin which is a powerful compound that has profound benefits on the human body. It acts as a natural anti-inflammatory. It relieves pain in arthritis patients. It helps in preventing and treating certain types of cancers. It boosts the immune system.

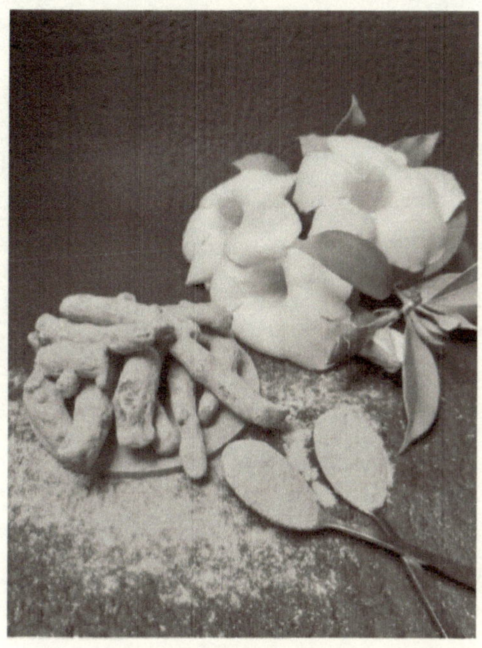

Picture 21: Turmeric

We can increase the bioavailability of curcumin by adding black pepper to it. Turmeric is available in its root form, powder, tablet, and capsule form. [62]

The simplest way to derive benefit from turmeric is by having turmeric milk or turmeric tea. Recipes are shared in the anti-inflammatory foods chapter.

Shatavari is also known as Asparagus racemosus. It has several health benefits.

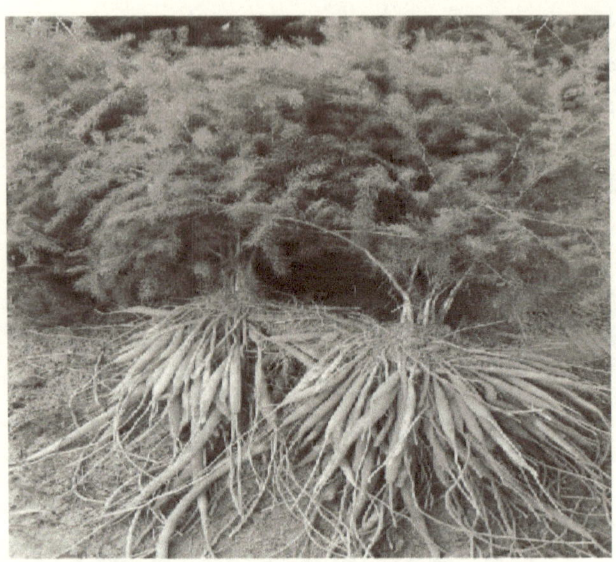

Picture 22: Shatavari

It is useful for gastric problems, inflammation, stress. It improves female health, stamina, and endurance. It relieves the menopausal symptoms. It balances the hormones. It's a female tonic for well-being and better stamina. It promotes quick recovery from sports injuries. [63]

Please consult a health practitioner before adding any of these herbs to one's daily diet.

Anti-Inflammatory Foods

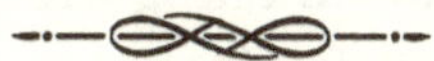

"There is an anti-dote provided by nature for everything. It's a self-sufficient ecosystem; all you need is to be part of it. "

What is Inflammation?

When the body is injured or ill, the immune system comes into action by increasing the blood flow to that area. The area gets puffy, red, and hot, which is called inflammation. Chronic inflammation is part of the immune system's natural response, but it attacks our body's tissue when the inflammation becomes chronic.

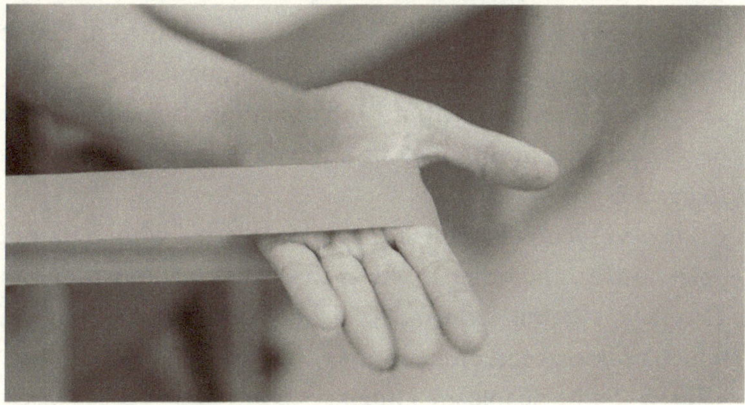

Picture 23: Inflammation

Inflammation is not only due to external injuries. Other factors contributing to inflammation are bad dietary habits, long-standing stress, lack of proper sleep, etc. Many athletes feel inflammation during their intense workouts or after an injury that lasts for a short period which is called acute inflammation. Long-standing inflammation due to eating wrong foods leads to chronic inflammation. This type of inflammation is the host of several diseases. [64]

Food that contributes to inflammation

- **Refined sugar-** Consuming a large amount of sugar causes inflammation.
- **Refined flour-** White flour encourages the growth of inflammation.
- **Trans fats-** Hydrogenated oils have trans fats that cause inflammation.
- **Processed foods-** Processed foods like burgers, pizza, packaged foods have high levels of preservatives and additives, which stimulate inflammation.
- **Omega 6 fatty acids-** Refined oils promote inflammation. There should be a balance in Omega 6 and Omega 3 fatty acids.
- **MSG-** MSG is Monosodium Glutamate that is used in Chinese and fast-food restaurants. It triggers inflammation.
- **Dairy-** It can result in chronic inflammation. If you feel gaseous or bloated after having milk or other dairy products, it is better to cut it down.
- **Processed meats-** Processed meats are injected with antibiotics, preservatives, and other additives that cause inflammation.
- **Excessive alcohol-** Too much alcohol damages the liver cells, which promotes inflammation.
- **Gluten-** Some people are gluten sensitive, like in celiac disease. Gluten causes inflammation for such people.

We should avoid the above foods to prevent and heal inflammation. [65]

Western medicine uses non-steroidal anti-inflammatory medications, corticosteroids which have long-term consequences. Always find holistic ways to deal with chronic inflammation. Make changes in the diet and incorporate anti-inflammatory foods to prevent or treat chronic inflammation.

Athletes who train for marathons, triathlons, and Ironman events get muscle and tissue tears, increasing the inflammation in the body. They need to choose an anti-inflammatory diet for smooth running. Avoid all the inflammatory foods mentioned above.

The anti-inflammatory diet is believed to fight inflammation in the body. It also increases immunity. These foods help release prostaglandins that help regulate the inflammatory response. Healing is facilitated through proper nutrition. [66]

Here is the list of top anti-inflammatory foods one can incorporate into their diet-

Pineapple

Digestive enzyme BROMELAIN is present in pineapple, which is used as an excellent anti-inflammatory agent. It supports faster recovery from injuries. Bromelain is present in a higher concentration in the stem of pineapple. It helps in digestion as it breaks down protein. It relieves the symptoms of indigestion, gas, heartburn. It is also beneficial for sinusitis, osteoarthritis, muscle soreness. It boosts immune health. Bromelain is administered for clinical applications in the treatment of inflammation and soft tissue injuries. [67]

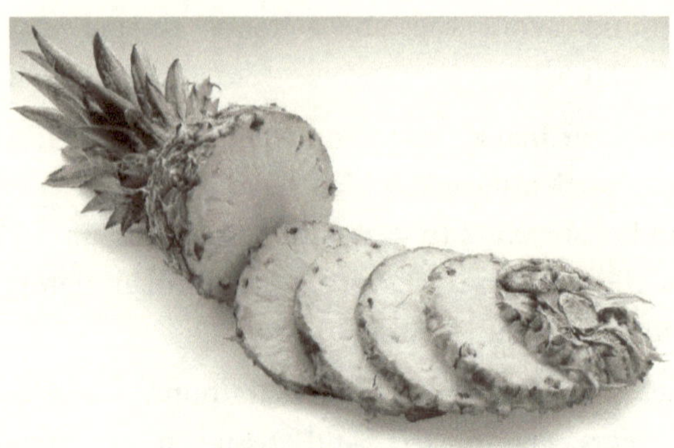

Picture 24: Pineapple

How to take bromelain- To reap the benefits of bromelain, have more pineapple and pineapple stem in your diet. To combat inflammation, we need large quantities of bromelain, and it may not be possible to eat large quantities of this fruit, so it's better to take it in a more concentrated form. Bromelain supplements are easily available. The dosage depends upon what it is being used for. If it is to be used as a digestive aid, it should be taken with meals, and for inflammation purposes, it should be taken on an empty stomach and between the meals.

People who are allergic to pineapple should not take bromelain supplements.

Turmeric comes from the root Curcuma longa, a member of the ginger family. Turmeric has Curcumin which is very effective in Inflammatory conditions. It reduces joint and muscle pain. It speeds up the healing process. Turmeric is rich in antioxidants. This spice accelerates the metabolism and fights against obesity. It also prevents certain cancer. Turmeric can be taken internally as well as can be applied externally on wounds. [68]

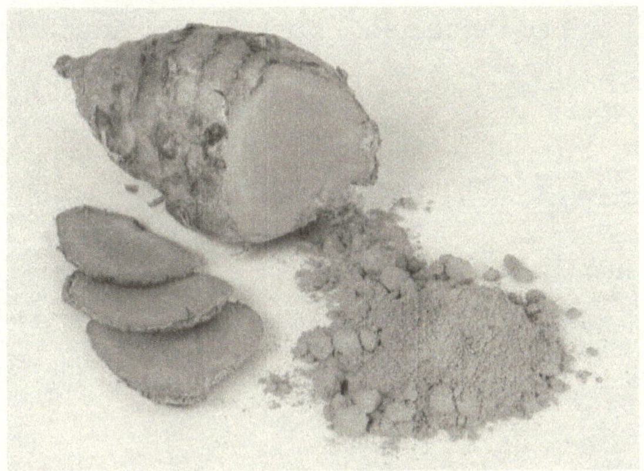

Picture 25: Turmeric

How to take turmeric- Best way to get turmeric's medicinal value is by taking it in the form of turmeric tea or latte. Below are some recipes-

Turmeric Tea

Prep: 15 mins; Cook: 10

Ingredients

- 1 tsp fresh grated turmeric
- 1 tsp fresh grated ginger
- ¼th tsp Cinnamon
- Juice of one lemon
- 1 tsp raw honey (optional)

Method

- Boil a cup of water along with grated turmeric and ginger.
- Cover and let it steep for 10 minutes.

- Strain it and add cinnamon, black pepper, honey, lemon juice, and enjoy.

Turmeric Milk

Prep: 10 mins; Cook: 10

Ingredients

- 1 tsp fresh grated turmeric
- 1 cup milk
- Pinch of black pepper
- 1 tsp ghee

Method

- Boil milk and turmeric for 7-8 minutes.
- Strain the milk and add ghee and pepper.

Note: The best time to drink turmeric milk is at night.

Turmeric Latte

Prep: 10 mins; Cook: 10

Ingredients

- 1 tsp fresh grated turmeric
- 1 tsp fresh grated ginger
- ¼th tsp Cinnamon
- Pinch of black pepper
- ¼th cup coconut milk
- 1 tsp raw honey (Optional)

Method

- Boil a mug of water along with crushed/grated turmeric and ginger for 5-6 minutes.
- Strain it and add the rest of the ingredients.
- Do not heat it after adding honey.
- Sip it while it's still warm.

Beets- Beets have an excellent anti-inflammatory property. It has fiber, phytonutrients which help in reducing inflammation. It lowers blood pressure. Beets have nitrates, which, when consumed, is converted into nitric oxide, which is beneficial for athletes. It increases the workout stamina, thereby improves athletic performance. [69]

Beets can be eaten with their greens. Have it in the form of salad, juice, sauté, or steam. If raw beets result in digestive troubles, then have them steamed. Fermented beets can also be eaten to reduce oxidative stress on the body. Fermented beets have probiotics that increase the good gut microbes.

People who are prone to kidney stones should take beets in limited quantities.

Ginger- Ginger works as a good anti-inflammatory drug. Ginger contains Gingerol, which has medicinal properties. It reduces muscle soreness and pain. It's also used to treat nausea and indigestion. It helps in lowering blood sugar and cholesterol.

Ginger can be taken in the form of ginger tea, or one can have it raw. For ginger tea, boil 2 cups of water add 1 tsp grated ginger root. Boil it for 5-6 minutes. Have it lukewarm. The other way of eating ginger is to grate it, sprinkle some lemon juice, and have it before meals.

Walnuts- Walnuts are high in Omega 3 fatty acids, which helps the body fight inflammation and lowers heart disease risk.

It helps in relieving symptoms of arthritis. It may help in preventing certain cancers. Walnuts strengthen the immune system and help improve memory. [70]

Soak 2 walnuts overnight and have it in the morning.

Dark leafy greens- Leafy greens contain healthy compounds that help reduce inflammation. Greens are a highly alkaline food, and inflammation can thrive only in an acidic environment. Everyone should consume greens daily. There are various ways to consume greens in salad, juice, soup, and saute. [71]

Cruciferous Vegetables- Cruciferous vegetables are full of nutrients and alkaline, helping the body eliminate inflammation. Examples of cruciferous vegetables are cabbage, cauliflower, mustard greens, turnip, kale, broccoli, brussels sprouts, etc.

These vegetables can be enjoyed in many forms like steaming, sautéing, boiling, and fermenting. [72]

Flaxseed- Flaxseed contain antioxidant and anti-inflammatory properties. It is a good source of Omega-3 fatty acids. The Omega-3 fatty acids are present inside the seeds, and to get the full benefits, they should be ground. [73]

You can add the ground flaxseeds to paranthas, dosas, soups, salads, fresh juices, desserts. Flaxseed oil is also easily available.

Sweet Potatoes- Sweet potatoes boost the immune system. It's high in vitamins and minerals. It has a lot of benefits for athletes as it provides a good amount of energy. It is also a very good pre-workout food. Sweet potatoes have phytonutrients that help in reducing inflammation. It can be eaten by baking or boiling.

Omega -3 fatty acids - Eating foods rich in Omega -3 fatty acids like walnuts, chia seeds, fish, cod liver oil, flaxseeds are associated with low levels of inflammatory markers.

Organic raw honey- Organic raw honey acts as an anti-bacterial and anti-inflammatory.

Coenzyme Q10 is also known as COQ10 or Ubiquinol, which our body produces naturally, but with age and other health-related factors, its production decreases. CoQ10 is required by every single cell in the body. CoQ10 is involved in energy production and also anti-inflammatory. It's good to treat heart problems, High blood pressure, High cholesterol, Chronic fatigue syndrome, and Parkinson's disease. [74]

For athletes, it increases stamina, decreases fatigue, and enhances recovery time. [75]

CoQ10 rich foods are free-range chicken, fish, eggs, sesame seeds, broccoli, and spinach. CoQ10 is present in these foods, but athletes who are over 40 should take it in a supplement form also, as due to age and oxidative stress, their body needs it for more energy production and proper blood flow. It's a beneficial supplement for endurance sports. Due to heavy training, there is a reduction of COQ10. Thereby, athletes need to take it in a supplementation form. It should be taken in the dosage of 200-300 mg for 2 - 6 weeks before the athletic event to enhance physical performance. The right dosage and the period depends upon several factors. Consult a doctor/dietician for the exact dosage and time frame.

Boswellia Serrata (Guggul/Shallaki)- The active ingredient boswellic acid found in guggul/shallaki is a powerful anti-inflammatory.

It reduces joint inflammation as well as neuroinflammation of the brain. It helps in sprains, strains, tendonitis, bursitis, osteoarthritis, rheumatoid arthritis, gout, IBD, fibromyalgia. It increases the blood supply to inflamed joints and helps to shrink the inflamed tissues. In Ayurveda, guggul is being used for a long to treat inflammatory diseases. [76]

If you have inflammation, the best time to take anti-inflammatory food is in the morning when the stomach is empty or in the day before taking meals when the stomach is nearly empty.

The best time to take turmeric milk is thirty minutes before bedtime.

Here are the few combination drinks you can have to prevent or treat inflammation-

- Pineapple, ginger juice
- Turmeric tea
- Turmeric latte
- Apple cider vinegar drink- Mix ½ cup water with 1 tablespoon ACV and 1tsp of honey.
- Green smoothie- 1cup spinach, 1inch ginger, half lemon
- Ginger lemonade- Take 1 tsp grated ginger. Boil for few minutes. Cool it and add 1 tsp lemon juice, 1 tsp honey, and 1 cup water.

You can incorporate a variety of anti-inflammatory foods throughout the day.

Micronutrients

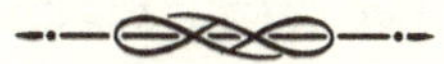

"Take care of the pennies, and the pounds will take care of themselves, the same rule applies to nutrients too, take care of the micros, and the macros will take care of themselves."

Micronutrients are nutrients that are needed in small quantities. Micronutrients play an important role in energy production, bone health, minimizing fatigue, helps in recovering muscle cramps, and better endurance performance. Intense or long workouts increase the loss of minerals through sweat. Greater intake of micronutrients may be required as per the body's needs due to endurance workouts.

Micronutrients are divided into two categories

Minerals and Vitamins

Macrominerals- Ca, Mg, Ph, Na, K

Trace minerals – Zn, Se, Co, Fe, Chromium

The human body requires both macro and trace minerals to maintain optimum health.

Calcium

Calcium is one of the most important minerals for athletes. It is important for healthy bones and teeth. Female athletes are highly prone to calcium deficiency. Calcium exertion may be increased with high-intensity training. It is important for a strong skeletal system and is also required for muscle contraction. Calcium gets absorbed in the body in the presence of Vitamin D. When there is a deficiency of Vitamin D, calcium is not bioavailable. If there is not enough calcium intake, then calcium is drawn from the bones, and bones get brittle, thereby increasing the chances of getting fractured during run injury.

The deficiency of calcium causes osteoporosis. It also leads to abnormal heart rhythms, muscle cramps. Deficiency may be due to various factors like not taking adequate calcium, certain diseases where calcium doesn't get absorbed properly, medications that hinder calcium absorption, hormonal disturbances in females, and Vitamin D deficiency.

Calcium-rich foods are milk, milk products, green leafy vegetables, sesame seeds, chia seeds, almonds, limestone.

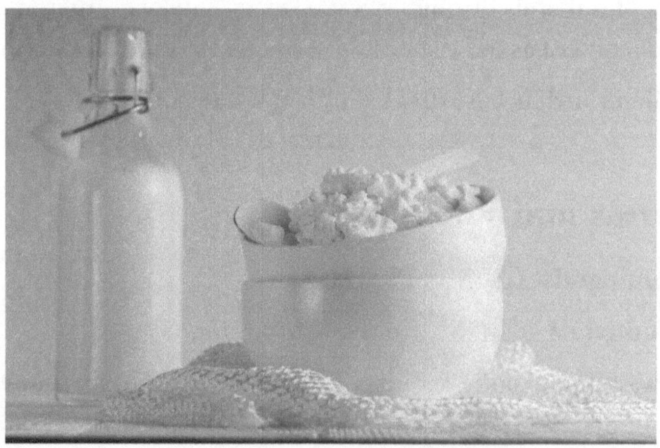

Picture 26: Dairy products

Recommended daily allowance (RDA) of Calcium - 1000 mg for adult men and women. Women older than 50 and men older than 70 years should take 1200mg daily.

Magnesium

Magnesium is essential for muscle relaxation. It helps in normal muscle, and nerve function, maintains the glucose level required for bones' formation, and improves sleep quality. Even a minimal Mg deficiency impairs athletic performance. For muscle cramps, magnesium and potassium help in fast recovery. It is an essential mineral for the human body and very beneficial for athletes. Magnesium comes in many forms like magnesium citrate, oxide, glycinate, sulfate, lactate, taurate. Magnesium citrate and oxide cause diarrhea at times; hence we recommend magnesium glycinate or taurate works.

Physically active individuals may have higher magnesium requirements for optimal performance. Magnesium also helps in reducing the accumulation of lactic acid.

Magnesium-rich foods are almonds, cashews, figs, pumpkin seeds, chia seeds, flaxseeds, dark chocolate, wheat, barley, oats, buckwheat, leafy greens, black beans, banana, Epsom salt for external spray.

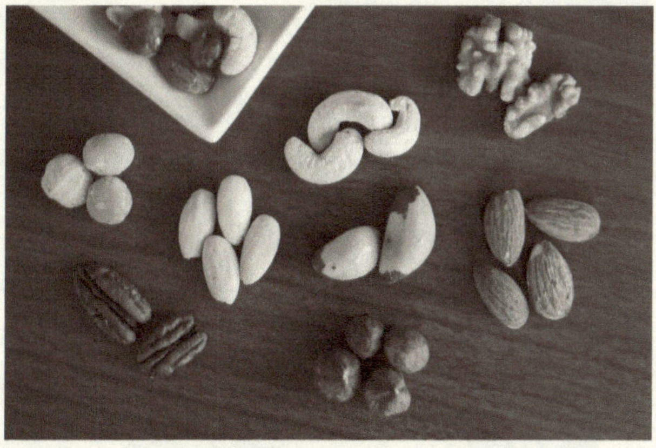

Picture 27: Nuts and Seeds

RDA Of Magnesium- For adult men and women, it should be between 310mg to 420mg. It varies with age. The recommended intake for endurance athletes is 500 to 700 mg daily, depending upon the training levels.

Sodium and Potassium

Potassium and Sodium work together for muscle function. When muscle contracts, sodium enters the cell, and potassium leaves the cell. Sodium is required for muscle contractions, and it also acts as a volume regulator. Muscles relax well if potassium is adequate, but muscles don't relax properly if potassium is deficient. Sodium is present outside the cell, whereas potassium is inside the cell. Sodium and Potassium together maintain the electrolyte balance in the body. Potassium loss during exercise causes damage to muscle tissue. During endurance workouts, the potassium loss is 100 to 200 mg per hour. That's the reason we stress that if one is working out more than an hour, then plain water doesn't help; always replenish with electrolytes. Symptoms of sodium and potassium deficiencies are nausea, vomiting, muscle cramping, spasm, etc.

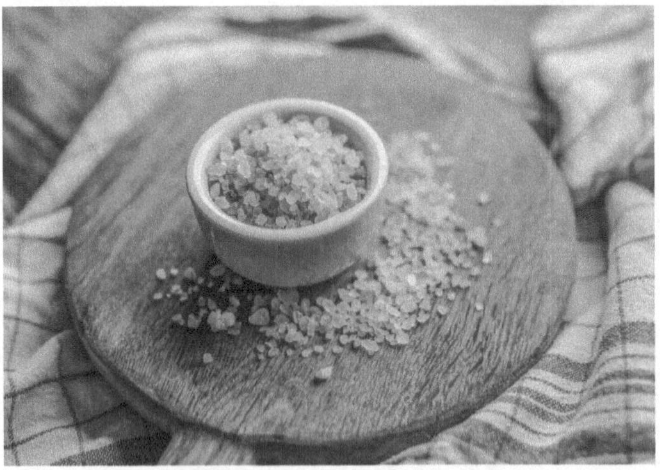

Picture 28: Himalayan pink salt

Examples **are** sea salt, banana, melons, dates, raisins, apricots, beans, chickpeas, peanuts, peas, sweet potato, pumpkin, coconut water.

RDA for sodium for adults- 1500mg. However, for athletes, it should increase depending on their workouts.

RDA for Potassium- 4700mg per day for adults. For endurance athletes additional 200-300 mg of potassium is required.

Chloride

Chloride is needed to keep the proper balance of body fluids. It's an important mineral and an electrolyte. Chloride moves freely in and out of the cells. Outside the cell, it is associated with sodium and inside the cell with potassium. Chloride is also part of hydrochloric acid in the stomach.

Chloride rich foods are sea salt, Seaweeds/Vegetables, rye

RDA for chloride- 2.0 – 2.3gms per day for adults

Iron

Iron is essential for athletic performance. Intense training increases the demand for iron. Without enough iron, oxygen cannot be used properly, which impairs athletic performance. Iron deficiency is a common problem in women athletes. Short of breath and feeling of tiredness call for a check of hemoglobin levels as iron is essential for hemoglobin formation. Anemia occurs if one does not have enough iron in the body. Take iron-rich foods. In case of higher deficiency, iron supplements or Intravenous iron will be required. Vitamin C enhances the absorption of iron.

Iron-rich foods are eggs, lean meats, beans, green leafy vegetables, black sesame seeds, pumpkin seeds, raisins. Eat vitamin C-rich food to get the maximum absorption of iron. The "Lucky Shakti Leaf" is a simple and effective way to improve iron levels in your body. It is produced by Lucky Iron Fish Enterprise, dedicated to solving iron deficiency and anemia. [77]

RDA- Men's- 8mg daily, Women's- 18mg daily.

Zinc

Zinc helps to keep the immune system healthy. Zinc is also needed for growth and development, acts as an antioxidant. Zinc aids in post-exertion tissue repair. It promotes wound healing and speeds up the recovery.

Zinc deficiency causes poor immunity, slower growth, delayed wound healing.

Zinc-rich foods are pumpkin seeds, hemp seeds, chickpeas, kidney beans, peanuts, almonds, cashews, seafood, whole grains, eggs, cocoa

RDA- Men's- 11mg daily, Women's- 8mg daily

Selenium

Selenium plays a critical role in thyroid hormone metabolism. It reduces the risk of cancer. It increases the antioxidant qualities. In athletes, it helps repair cellular damage.

The deficiency of selenium causes fatigue, muscle weakness, and a weak immune system.

Selenium rich foods are whole grains, eggs, lentils, oats, lean meat, fish, sunflower seeds, kidney beans, cashews, banana

RDA- 55 micrograms for adults

Vitamins

Vitamins are naturally occurring substances needed for many processes in the body. Vitamins prevent and treat diseases. Vitamins are either water-soluble or fat-soluble. Inadequate intake of any vitamin causes deficiency. It's better to take vitamins through the food.

Critical Vitamins

- Vitamin A
- Vitamin B- B1, B2, B3, B5, B6, B7, B9, B12
- Vitamin C
- Vitamin D
- Vitamin E
- Vitamin K
- All Vitamins are essential for overall well-being.

Vitamin A

This vitamin is essential for maintaining vision and plays an important role in the immune system. It helps in relieving inflammation. It prevents and treats certain types of cancers. **Vitamin A-rich foods are** sweet potato, Carrots, Pumpkin, Dark green leafy vegetables, Tomatoes, Mangoes, Papaya, egg yolks

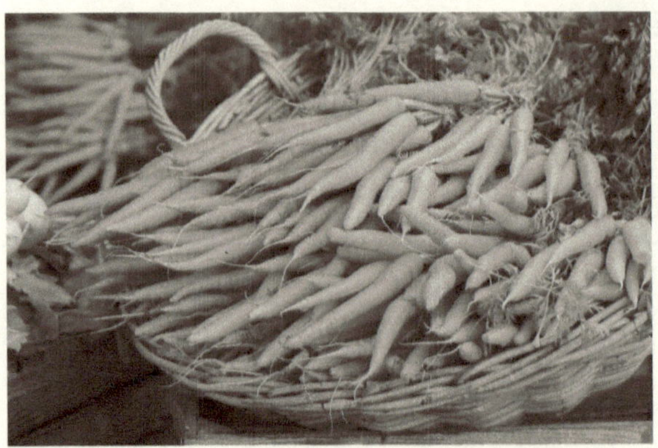

Picture 29: Vitamin A-rich foods

RDA for Vitamin A- 900 micrograms

Vitamin B1 (Thiamine) metabolizes food into energy.

RDA- 1.5mg

Vitamin B2 (Riboflavin) is important in the maintenance of tissues of the body. It is also required for proper development of the body.

RDA- 1.1mg

Vitamin B3 (Niacin) breaks down food into energy.

RDA- 20mg

Vitamin B5 (Pantothenic acid) has a role to play in several different biological processes.

RDA-10mg

Vitamin B6 (Pyridoxine) helps in metabolism and increases energy levels.

RDA- 2mg

Vitamin B7 (Biotin) cures nerve damage, hair fall, brittle nails.

RDA- 300 micrograms

Vitamin B9 (folate) is required for red blood formation. This vitamin is essential during early pregnancy to reduce congenital disabilities. It also reduces the high level of homocysteine.

RDA- 400 micrograms

Vitamin B 12 (Cobalamins) helps in maintaining the health of nerve cells. It supports healthy metabolism and digestion. It enables the body to produce red blood cells. If you are having low energy and get fatigued easily, do check your B12 levels as this vitamin converts the food into glucose which provides energy to the body. Lack of this vitamin causes chronic fatigue, mood swings, memory loss, dry skin, anemia. For some people, vitamin B12 does not get absorbed due to the lack of hydrochloric acid. In that case, it should be taken externally in the form of tablets or injections.

As all the B vitamins are water-soluble, it gets excreted in the urine. So, it should be consumed regularly. It doesn't get stored in the body.

Vitamin B rich foods are whole grains, leafy greens, legumes, milk, sunflower seeds, chicken, fish, liver, eggs

RDA- 6 micrograms

All these eight vitamins make up the so-called "B- complex."

Vitamin C (Ascorbic acid) increases immunity, plays a vital role in wound healing. Vitamin C helps to repair and regenerate tissues. It protects the body from various cancers. Vitamin C is water-soluble; our body doesn't store it. So, it's essential to take it daily.

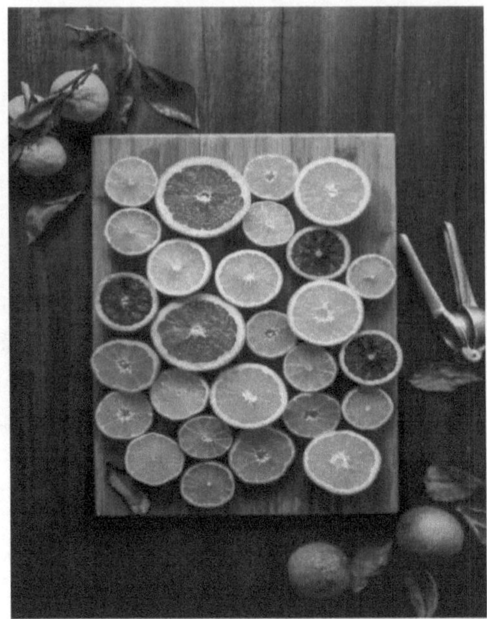

Picture 30: Vitamin C rich foods

Vitamin C rich foods are Oranges, lemons, pineapple, tomatoes, capsicum, guava, papaya.

RDA- 500mg

Vitamin D is also called the sunshine vitamin, which the body makes using sunlight. Vitamin D helps our body to absorb calcium. It promotes healthy bones. Sufficient vitamin D protects us from some cancers. It reduces the risk of diabetes.

Vitamin D is an essential nutrient for athletes. Athletes are at a higher risk of fractures, so it's critical to take this vitamin regularly. It also enhances athletic performance. Vitamin D deficiency causes muscle weakness, pain in the bones, osteoporosis, a higher risk of sports injuries, stress fractures.

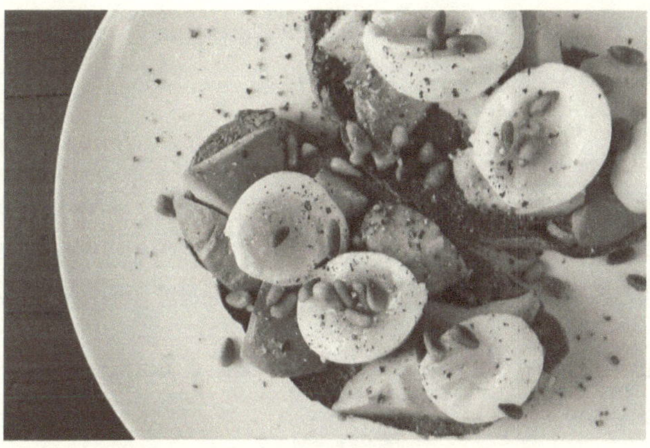

Picture 31: Vitamin D rich foods

Vitamin D-rich foods: Sunlight is the largest source of Vitamin D, fatty fish, fish oils, cod liver oil, egg yolk.

RDA- 35 micrograms daily

Vitamin E reduces free radical damage, helps fight inflammation, good for the heart, skin, and hair. It balances the hormones naturally. It strengthens the immune system. It helps in the prevention and treatment of cataracts. Aerobic athletes may have an increased need for vitamin E as their cells undergo oxidative damage.

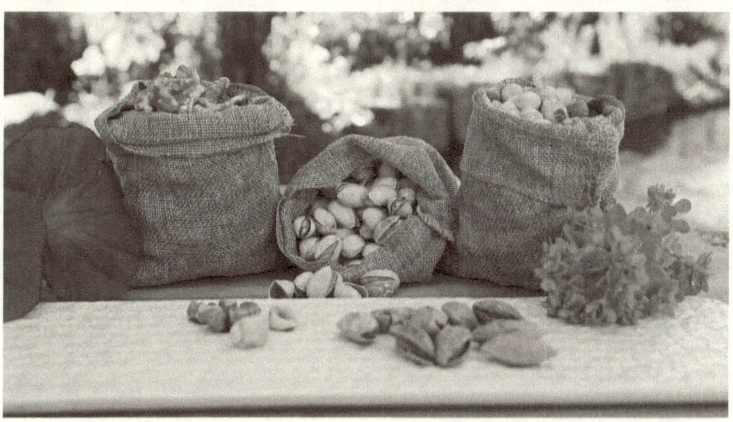

Picture 32: Vitamin E rich food

Vitamin E rich foods are almonds, peanuts, seeds, leafy greens, coconut oil, wheat germ, mango.

RDA- 22.4 IU

Vitamin K plays a vital role in blood clotting. This vitamin also prevents heart diseases and helps in bone building. Deficiency causes- increased bleeding, bruising, and heavy periods.

Vitamin K rich foods are Leafy greens, cucumbers, cauliflower, cabbage, eggs.

RDA- 70- 90 micrograms

Water-soluble vitamins are all the Vitamin B and Vitamin C. They are found in fruits, vegetables, and grains. They dissolve in water and get excreted in the urine, so we should get them regularly from our diet.

Fat-soluble vitamins are Vitamins A, D, E, and K. These vitamins are soluble in fats; that's why it's essential to include good fats in the diet. When someone eliminates one or more food groups from their diet, it can result in a deficiency of some vitamin or mineral. So, eat a well-balanced diet.

There are several ways to absorb or take these micronutrients and three means to transport these nutrients.

Oral- Vitamins and minerals can be gained by incorporating a variety of food sources. If you are deficient in some specific micronutrient, then consume those food sources which are rich in that vitamin or mineral.

If one cannot make it from food, supplements are also available in natural forms.

Transdermal Delivery- Some people get stomach upset by taking vitamins and minerals in a supplementation form. Another alternative is to enrich your body with these supplements through the skin. This is called transdermal technology. In this technology, the preparation is to be sprayed onto the skin.

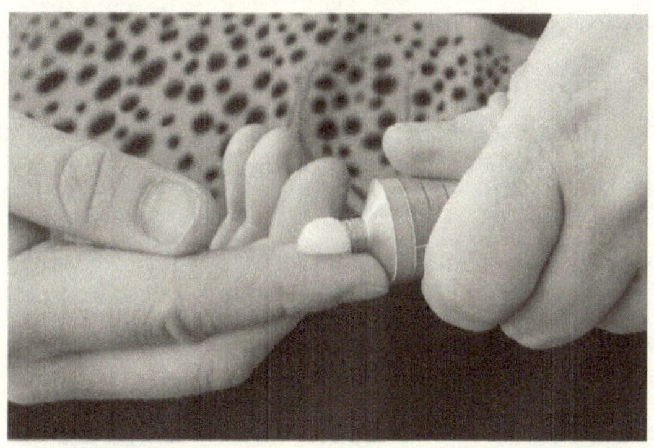

Picture 33: Transdermal delivery

Take the magnesium from magnesium oil spray or Epsom salt soak. Sprays, gels, creams are available for transdermal delivery of vitamins and minerals.

Intravenous- If one has an extreme deficiency that cannot be rectified from food, I.V. therapy works.

Intravenous Therapy

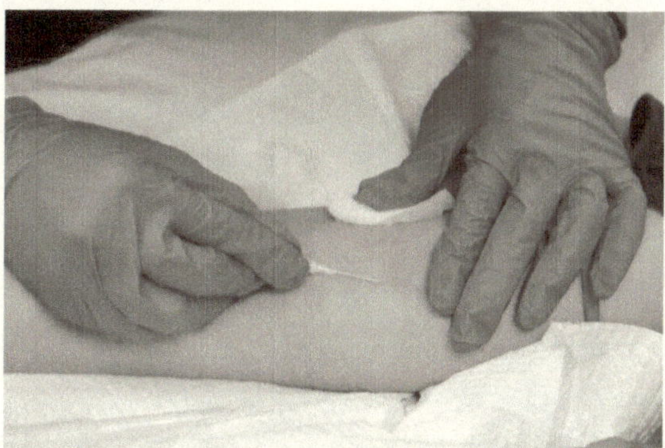

Picture 34: Intravenous therapy

Due to poor health of the gut or due to missing specific enzyme nutrients that don't get absorbed properly, replacements of vitamins and minerals can be achieved by I.V.

Recommended intakes of nutrients vary with age, sex, health conditions, pregnancy, and lactation. Endurance athletes need more of these nutrients. Consult a health care practitioner for one's requirements [78]

Endocrine System

"Chemical Locha" happens when you hurry, Worry and Curry. To keep your hormonal balance, replace the Hurry with being Thoughtful, the Worry with being Mindful, and the Curry with being Healthful. Be full to be vibrant."

The endocrine system consists of all the glands of the body, which work by secreting hormones into the bloodstream. These glands secrete hormones to regulate many functions in the human body. Hormones are chemicals that carry messages from one cell to another through the bloodstream. The hypothalamus, pituitary, and pineal gland are located in our brain. The thyroid and parathyroid are in our neck. The thymus gland is located in the middle of our chest. Then we have the pancreas, adrenals in the abdominal part and ovaries, testes in the pelvic region. The study of the endocrine system and its disorders is known as endocrinology. The endocrine system helps in growth, metabolism, reproduction, stress, emotional behavior. This system is responsible for regulating hunger, nutrient usage, absorption, and storage. The endocrine system uses blood vessels to deliver hormones. The glands must release the correct amount of hormones to maintain the balance. If they release less or more, it creates a hormonal imbalance. The functions of the Endocrine system are connected to the body's nutrition. Adequate nutrition is essential for the functioning of all these glands [79]

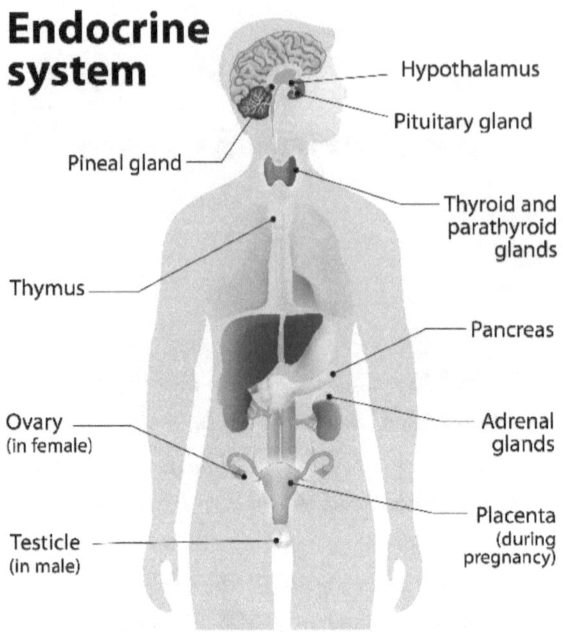

Picture 35: Endocrine System

Hypothalamus Gland

It is located inside the brain and maintains the body's internal balance. This gland helps in maintaining blood pressure, heart rate, temperature, body weight, appetite, sleep.

The main hormones secreted by the hypothalamus are corticotropin-releasing hormone, anti-diuretic hormone, growth hormone, oxytocin, prolactin, somatostatin, gonadotropin-releasing hormone.

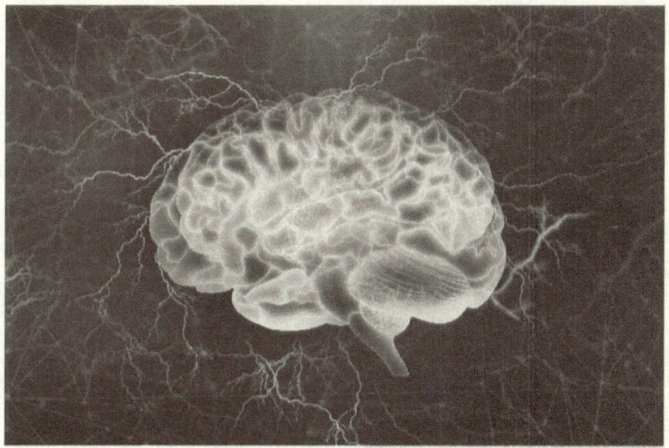

Picture 36: Brain

Pituitary Gland

It is called the master gland as it controls several hormones in the body. Hypothalamus gives a signal to the pituitary gland to stimulate or inhibit hormone production. The main hormones are follicle-stimulating hormone, growth hormone, luteinizing hormone, oxytocin, and adrenocorticotropic hormone.

Pineal Gland

The pineal gland makes melatonin which helps the body to sleep.

Thyroid and Parathyroid Glands

The thyroid gland and the parathyroid glands are in the base of the neck. These glands produce triiodothyronine (T3) and thyroxine (T4), calcitonin. These hormones have a vital function to perform in the body's metabolic rate and control the calcium ion levels in the blood. Hypothyroidism and hyperthyroidism conditions are due to less or more secretion of thyroid hormones.

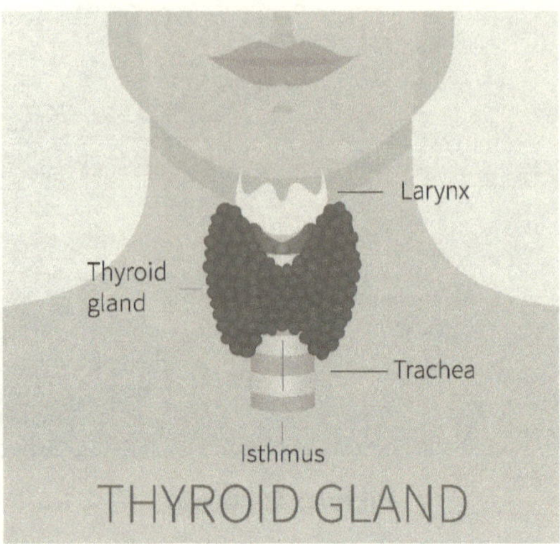

Picture 37: Thyroid Gland

We all are unique in the functioning of the hormones. It's better to go for thyroid panel tests that include

- TSH
- Free T3
- Free T4
- Calcitonin
- Thyroid antibodies

Relationship between hypothyroidism and weight

When the body doesn't make enough thyroid hormone, it results in hypothyroidism leading to a slowdown in metabolism. There are salt and water retention, which results in weight gain and bloating. An underactive thyroid does not burn as much energy as it stores, thus leading to weight gain. The more severe hypothyroidism is, the more weight one gains. It's essential to find out the cause of hypothyroidism, such as if it's Hashimoto's or thyroiditis. [80]

A person with hypothyroidism should eat a high-fiber diet that has fewer calories. The diet should contain lots of veggies, fresh fruits, lean proteins, and healthy carbs. Cardio, strength training, and HIIT are a must for weight loss.

Natural ways to maintain thyroid health

Thyroid medication may cause some side effects like nausea, vomiting, palpitations, and mood swings. Thyroid problems can be managed by changing diet and lifestyle. If one suffers from thyroid, then cabbage, broccoli, cauliflower, bok choy should be avoided in their raw form. If they are cooked, they can be taken in moderate quantities. Uncooked cruciferous vegetables disrupt thyroid functions, and such veggies are called" Goitrogens." Stay clear of high sugar and processed foods. Include more green, yellow and orange foods. Take lean protein and fatty fish. Include iodized salt and sea vegetables in the diet. Take supplements of Vitamin D and selenium. Cold-pressed coconut oil helps in hypothyroidism. Ujjayi pranayama is very useful in combating thyroid disorders. Several ayurvedic medicines can be taken as per doctor consultation. [81]

Pancreas

It makes the hormones insulin and glucagon. Diabetes is caused due to imbalances in the production of insulin. Insulin is released in the body when there are high blood glucose levels. Glucagon is released in the body when there are low blood glucose levels. Insulin and glucagon need to work in partnership with each other to keep the blood glucose levels in a balanced state. Glucagon is the hormone that promotes the breakdown of glycogen to glucose in the liver. Insulin is required when there is hyperglycemia, and glucagon is required in hypoglycemia. In other words, glucagon has the opposite effect of insulin.

Adrenal Glands

The adrenal glands are also called suprarenal glands, as they are located above the kidneys.

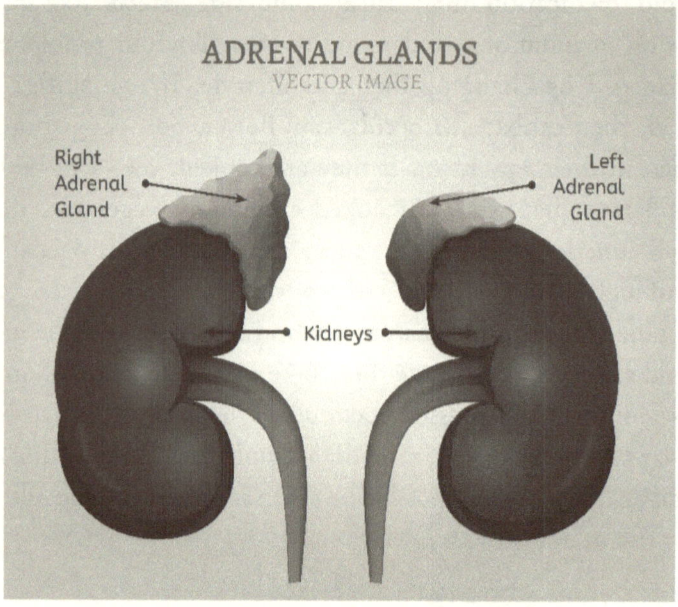

Picture 38: Adrenal Glands

The hormones they produce are cortisol, aldosterone, adrenaline. These hormones help in regulating metabolism, helps control blood pressure, helps the body to react to stress.

Adrenal Fatigue

"Adrenal fatigue is a group of related signs and symptoms that results when the adrenal glands function below the necessary levels," is described by James Wilson, who is an expert in alternative medicine. He says people with adrenal fatigue feel tired all the time, don't sleep well and crave salty foods. If you have long-standing stress, adrenal fatigue sets in. The theory is that chronic stress wears down the adrenal glands so that they produce fewer stress hormones when stressors continue. Common symptoms are fatigue, trouble falling asleep, body aches, loss of hair, poor digestion.

According to Ayurveda, adrenal fatigue is due to Vata vitiation. It's crucial to pacify Vata.

Adopting healthy lifestyle measures is highly beneficial in Adrenal fatigue.

- Follow daily routine (dincharya) as mentioned in the Ayurveda chapter.
- Detoxification is necessary to clean the ama (toxins) as per body needs.
- Inculcate more anti-inflammatory foods
- Focus on whole foods
- Take probiotics
- Eliminate or reduce stress
- Exercise regularly
- Refrain from processed and stale food
- Ayurvedic herbs Brahmi, ashwagandha, shilajit, yastimadhu helps in clearing adrenal fatigue.

Ovaries

Ovaries in women make estrogen and progesterone.

Estrogen is the primary female sex hormone. Estrogen plays a role in the reproductive system. Women who are overweight have more fat cells that produce excess estrogen in the body. High levels of estrogen increase belly fat. Excess estrogen causes various health issues like PCOS, ovarian cysts, uterine fibroids, irregular periods, heavy bleeding. It is also the risk factor for ovarian cancer, endometrial cancer, and breast cancer.

Symptoms of excess estrogen

- Weight gain- Excess estrogen causes accumulation of fat on the waist, hips, and thighs.
- Digestive issues- Burping, bloating and fullness are the common signs.
- Breast tenderness- Soreness or swollen breasts could be due to excess estrogen.
- Irregular periods- Heavy or scanty periods are related to hormonal changes.
- Mood swings, depression, anxiety, headaches, loss of sex drive, and fatigue are common due to excess estrogen.

Ways to lower estrogen levels naturally

- Include a lot of cruciferous vegetables in your diet like cauliflower, cabbage, broccoli, turnips.
- Eat organic produce. Include more dark leafy greens.
- Estrogen is excreted by the bowl. Get more fiber in your diet. Eat a diet rich in insoluble fiber. Take Triphala at night to clear the bowls.
- Avoid processed, high-fat and sugary foods.
- Avoid plastic bottles and containers.
- Avoid soy and soy products.
- Intermittent fasting helps a lot to get rid of excess estrogen.
- Pay attention to liver health, as the liver removes excess estrogen from the body. Detoxification of the liver is crucial. Stay clear from caffeine and alcohol.

- Regular exercise is a must. Lose excess body fat and weight.
- Twisted and abdominal yoga asanas help a lot in gynecological issues.
- Reduce stress.
- Aim for 7-8 hours of sleep

Testes

Testes make testosterone in men.

Endocrine diseases result when a gland produces too little or too much of a hormone.

Common endocrine disorders are

Hypothyroidism, hyperthyroidism, diabetes, hypoglycemia, osteoporosis, PCOD, adrenal insufficiency, tumors

Gastrointestinal hormones

Gut hormones are a group of hormones secreted by endocrine cells in the stomach, pancreas, and small intestine. These hormones regulate many functions in the body. Most of these hormones are released after a meal for digestion and absorption of nutrients.

Gastrin is a hormone released by the stomach. When we eat food, gastrin tells the stomach to release hydrochloric acid. This acid breaks the food, and then the food moves to the intestine.

Secretin is the hormone released by the duodenum. Its primary function is to neutralize stomach acid.

Cholecystokinin (CCK)is produced in the duodenum and jejunum. It responds to protein and fats. It stimulates the gall bladder to contract and empty.

Motilin participates in controlling muscle contractions in the stomach as well as in the small intestine.

We have hunger hormones Ghrelin and Leptin. It's a must to get to know about these hormones for people who are into weight loss.

Ghrelin is made in the stomach, and this hormone makes us feel hungry. When it is secreted in the stomach, it sends a signal to the brain that causes us to feel hungry. In other words, ghrelin increases appetite. Ghrelin levels go up before mealtimes and go down after eating the meal. When the body is under stress, ghrelin is released, and that's the reason people tend to eat more when they are under stress. Ghrelin contributes to weight gain.

Leptin is a hormone that decreases appetite, so it is called "Starvation Hormone." Leptin is made up of fat cells, so it is called fat hormone. Leptin signals the brain that the body has energy, so food is not required. When the leptin level is high, hunger is reduced. In an overweight person, there is "leptin resistance," which means when they eat, the brain isn't getting the signal of fullness. That's why they keep eating more. Several factors lead to leptin resistance. Those factors are a sedentary lifestyle, eating processed food, under constant stress.

Obesity results from eating too much, little physical activity, hormone imbalance, unmonitored usage of medicines, and genetics. So, work on all the factors to see significant results.

The question arises, what dietary changes should we make to control these two hormones to get the ideal weight?

- Eat a well-balanced, nutrient-dense diet. Consume healthy fats.
- Have your last meal before sunset. It should be light.

- Green Coffee contains bioactive 'Chlorogenic acid' that has shown anti-obesity and anti-inflammatory effects.[82]
- Stay away from processed foods, bad fats. Snack on cucumber salads whenever you have hunger pangs.
- Have more fiber in the diet.
- Regular exercise is a must, especially high-intensity interval training. Exercise can be done at any time of the day, but mornings are the best as it helps in ghrelin production.
- Good sleep and stress management is equally responsible for balancing these hormones.
- Focus on breathing exercises will improve your metabolism. A few examples are Kapalbhati, Bastrika pranayam, Ujjayai pranayam, Agnisar pranayam and Nadi shodhan pranayam.

How pollution affects the Endocrine system

Due to pollutants, the functioning of the endocrine system gets disrupted. These pollutants include plastics, perfumes, lotions, cosmetics, industrial chemicals, pesticides, and herbicides. These are called endocrine disruptors. [83]

All of us breathe polluted air every day. These pollutants interfere with the actions of hormones as well as interfere with the activity of enzymes. This endocrine disruption may develop in the fetus itself, which can lead to metabolic disorders. These days, there is a decrease in the age of puberty. This could be due to endocrine hormone disturbance. Endocrine disrupters like chemicals, pollutants may cause early puberty.

Polluted air is inhaled from the nose and damages the lungs. From there, it goes to the bloodstream and damages other parts of the body too. When athletes run on the roads, they get exposed to various gases like carbon monoxide, dust, smoke, and pollen.

When food and water are stored in plastic boxes, plastic bottles, plastic wraps, and aluminum foils, chemicals leach from the package into food, contributing to chronic diseases.

How athletes can avoid these endocrine disrupters-

- Try to run in the early hours and avoid congested areas.
- Practice nasal breathing. Breathe in through your nose, breathe out through your nose. Keep your mouth closed.
- During running or cycling, always wear nose filters or use pollution masks, dust masks. Nowadays, we are using a mask for the COVID-19 situation, which stands helpful against pollution too.
- Avoid plastic bottles. Use stainless steel bottles or copper bottles or use silicon sippers.
- After training sessions, always wash your hands properly.
- Refrain from eating canned food. Choose fresh produce.
- Eat organic, local foods.
- Avoid plastic boxes or plastic packaging for food.
- Use fragrance-free natural-made cosmetics.
- Stay away from chemical cleaners. Instead of that, use lemon, vinegar, baking soda.

Testosterone

Testosterone is a hormone produced by both men and women though men produce in a large amount, which is the reason why men have more muscle mass than women. A fair amount of testosterone levels are needed for optimum performance in athletes, and it is also necessary to maintain their energy levels. Testosterone declines with age, poor health, and poor diet. If a person over trains, then testosterone levels drop. It also drops for people who take a very low-fat diet.

Normal levels of testosterone in Men: 350-1198 ng/dl

Women: 7- 48 ng/dl

How overtraining reduces testosterone levels in athletes

Overtraining is one of the biggest reasons for the testosterone drop-in in athletes. Overtraining increases oxidative stress and also raises cortisol levels. It decreases immunity. Increased cortisol means more stress, which the body is not able to flush out. [84]

Signs of reduced testosterone

- Reduced muscle mass.
- Reduced bone mass.
- Low sex drive.
- Increased body fat.
- Mood swings.
- Sleep disturbances.
- Tiredness.

Here are some natural ways to raise the testosterone levels.

- Do not over-train. Discuss with your coach about the training plan.
- Include good fat in your diet.
- Include B- complex vitamins in your diet.
- Sufficient Vitamin D and magnesium.
- Stay clear from sugar and refined foods.
- Avoid processed packaged foods.
- Regular endurance running, resistance training also increases this hormone.
- Sleep well.

- Minimize stress by practicing meditation and deep breathing.
- Foods that increase testosterone levels are eggs, apples, pineapples, pomegranate, cruciferous vegetables, spinach, oysters, garlic, walnuts, brazil nuts, fish oil, dark chocolate and coconut oil.
- Avoid Phyto-estrogens, which increases estrogen in the body, which in turn decreases testosterone. Examples are soy and soy products, flaxseeds, fenugreek seeds, licorice. These foods have many other benefits; however, avoid them two weeks before the run event.
- Alcohol- Too much alcohol decreases testosterone. It's a good idea to give up or limit alcohol consumption.
- Refined oils- All kinds of heavily processed refined oils diminish testosterone levels. Switch to cold-pressed oils.
- Too many sugary, trans fat, and refined foods like cakes, desserts, donuts, bread should be at a bare minimum.
- Mint- Mint reduces testosterone production.

Effects of alcohol on the Endocrine system

Alcohol abuse disrupts the functioning of the endocrine system. Alcohol intoxication induces several diseases in the body like hormonal imbalance, immune dysfunction, cardiovascular diseases, impair reproductive functions, blood pressure, calcium malabsorption. [85]

Effects of drinking alcohol on athletes

Heavy drinking is common after athletic events. Avoid post-race binge drinking. [86] Try to eliminate them due to the following negative effects

- Alcohol is a diuretic; it dehydrates the body.
- It disrupts the sleep pattern.

- It is just empty calories with zero nutrition. These calories are stored around the stomach area, known as a beer belly.
- Alcohol imbalances the glucose levels, and one craves to eat more sugary foods.
- It interferes with protein synthesis, as a result, slows down recovery.
- It raises blood pressure.
- After running, muscles are inflamed, and alcohol consumption adds up more inflammation.
- Inability to absorb essential nutrients.

There is no doubt that alcohol negatively affects performance. Alcohol is an endocrine disrupter.

Healing Foods

"Your bio-mechanical machine requires periodic servicing and nature provides all the tools to set it right, the service station is your kitchen, not the pharma."

The human body can be afflicted by several diseases. Below is a compiled list of the most common ailments. There is a specific treatment for every person as per their symptoms and body type. However, below are some generalized remedies.

Cough and Cold is a common problem that occurs in the rainy season and during winters.

- Stay hydrated- drink plenty of water and other homemade beverages.
- Gargling- Gargle with warm water mixed with salt.
- Steam inhalation helps a lot.
- Apply Eucalyptus oil on your handkerchief and put it under your pillow while sleeping.
- Ginger helps a lot in this condition. It removes the phlegm. Boil ginger in a cup of water and add lemon and honey once it is a little cool. Sip it slowly.
- Turmeric milk helps in boosting immunity and fights infection. Drink turmeric milk thirty minutes before sleeping.
- Drink tulsi tea.
- For bad cough, chew licorice (mulethi) stick.

Gas and Bloating is a common problem faced by many, including athletes. Making some changes in the diet can easily combat this problem.

- Take small bites and chew the food well.
- Be mindful while eating.
- Chew grated ginger with rock salt and lemon before the meal.
- Chew 1 tsp of fennel seeds after meals.
- Incorporate more probiotics into the diet.
- Drink Buttermilk with asafetida after lunch.
- Hingwashtak Churan ½ tsp twice a day with warm water.

Headache/Migraine is a common and unbearable condition that many people deal with. Certain food intake causes headaches. Try to find out if there are any food intolerances. Usually, MSG, ice cream, chocolates, nuts cause headaches. If it is food-related, then make a food log and see which food causes headaches and avoid that. Sometimes digestive issues like gas, acidity also causes headache. Hormonal imbalances also cause headaches.

Here are some tips to prevent and treat headaches

- Get a head massage done regularly.
- Drink plenty of water.
- During the headache, apply some ice pack on the forehead.
- Reduce stress. Regular Pranayama helps.
- Use Essential oils roll-ons rather than take any medication. [87]

If headaches are persistent or headaches and some other symptoms appear quite often, seek help from a health practitioner.

A sprain is one of the most common injuries for athletes. It's an injury in which ligaments twist, which causes pain and swelling.

- Apply an ice pack to the inflamed area for the first 48hours. Do this for 20 minutes every 3-4 hours.
- Epsom salt- If there is no open wound, one can soak the twisted part in Epsom salt water for 20-30 minutes. The magnesium helps reduce soreness and relaxes the muscles.
- Wrap the crepe bandage to reduce swelling
- Give rest to that area
- Keep the injured part elevated above the heart.
- Take more anti-inflammatory food, which aids in healing

Toothache is irritating and, if not treated on time, leads to radiating pain.

- Saltwater rinse is an effective treatment for toothache. Mix ½ tsp of salt in warm water and swish it inside the mouth for few minutes.
- Oil pulling is an extremely beneficial treatment for toothache. It even prevents cavities. Please refer to the chapter of "Ayurveda" for more details.
- Dab a few drops of clove oil onto a cotton ball and apply it to the affected area.
- Use neem brush stick regularly to ward off infections.
- Mix ½ tsp of mustard oil and ¼th tsp of salt and apply this on teeth. Do this regularly to prevent toothache.

Diabetes Excess sugar in the blood causes diabetes. When there is too much sugar in the blood, the body tries to make extra insulin. However, the pancreas cannot keep up with the high demands. So, the glucose levels go high in the blood.

- Bitter gourd juice- Drink 20-30 ml bitter gourd juice on an empty stomach.

- Fenugreek seeds- Have sprouted fenugreek seeds or soak 1tsp seeds in water and leave it overnight. Drink this water in the morning and chew the seeds.
- Cinnamon powder- Add cinnamon powder in water and take this regularly.
- Indian Gooseberry- Include Amla in your diet.
- Eat food that has a low glycemic index.
- Take Triphala at night.
- Jamun and curry leaves help a lot in reducing blood sugar levels.
- Exercise for 30-60 minutes a day.

Hypertension affects millions of people. Most of the time, there are no symptoms and puts you at an increased risk for chronic kidney disease, heart disease, heart failure, and stroke, among other things; that is the reason it is called "Silent Killer." High blood pressure can easily be managed by following few remedies

- Regular exercise is one of the best ways to reduce blood pressure.
- Reduce the consumption of salt.
- Chew 2-3 garlic cloves on an empty stomach.
- Arjun chaal or capsules are tonics for the heart.
- Sipping 2 cups of hibiscus tea every day lowers the pressure.
- Beetroot juice has relaxing effects on blood vessel linings.
- Have more potassium-rich foods like banana, melons, papaya, orange, beets, raisins, coconut water.

Athlete's Foot is a fungal infection that affects the skin of the feet. People who wear sweaty shoes and socks for long are prone to this infection. It is highly contagious. Gyms, swimming pool areas, locker rooms are the commonly found area where fungus thrives.

- Wash your feet every day with soap and water and pat dry.
- Take ½ cup apple cider vinegar and 3 cups of warm water in a bucket. Soak your feet for 15-20 minutes. Pat dry.
- Mix few drops of tea tree oil in coconut oil and apply it to the feet.
- Make a paste using baking soda and water and apply this paste to the affected area. Wash after few minutes and apply coconut oil.
- Take probiotics internally, which increases the good gut bacteria that fight the fungal infection.
- Boil some neem leaves in water and soak feet in this water for 15 minutes and pat dry.

The diseases given above are prevalent. If left untreated, they can have severe complications. It is vital to treat them naturally. Do consult a medical practitioner before starting any remedy.

Tissue Salts

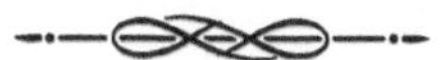

"Our body is made up of millions of cells that communicate with each other through chemical signaling. To keep this network running, you need to be a good service provider."

Tissue salts are also called Dr. Schuessler's biochemical cell salts. Tissue salts are made up of the same minerals that are found in soil and rocks. Due to pollution, pesticide, and fungicide usage, the soil is deprived of minerals. This is the reason for not getting the right amount of minerals from our food. Secondly, due to stress, heavy metals, electronic radiation, our body does not absorb the nutrients from food. Tissue salts are the best way to get the right amount of minerals. [88]

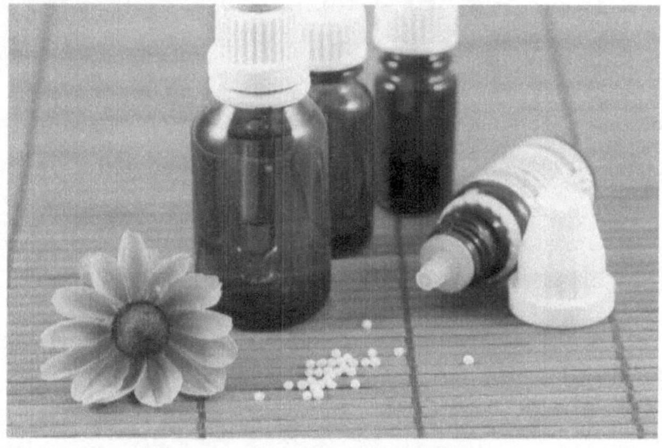

Picture 39: Tissue Salts

- ***Calc Flour Tissue Salt*** People with cracked skin, brittle nails, weak connective tissues can use tissue salt.
- ***Calc Phos Tissue Salt*** People with teeth and bone problems can use this.
- ***Calc Sulph Tissue Salt*** Act as a blood purifier and can be used for purulent infections.
- ***Ferr Phos Tissue Salt*** Anti-inflammatory, oxygen supplier to the cells, useful in anemia.
- ***Kali Mur tissue Salt*** Used in tonsillitis, sore throat, and other sluggish conditions. Kali Mur is potassium chloride that helps to form fibrin.
- ***Kali Phos Tissue Salt*** Useful for conditions related to nerves/headaches/nervous tension.
- ***kali Sulf tissue Salt*** Useful for catarrhal problems and athlete's foot.
- ***Mag Phos Tissue Salt*** Useful for runner's cramps, pains, twitching's and spasms.
- ***Nat Mur Tissue Salt*** Acts as a water distributor.
- ***Nat Phos Tissue Salt*** Maintains the acid-base balance, acts as an acid neutralizer.
- ***Nat Sulph Tissue Salt*** Helpful in liver problems and digestion.
- ***Silicea Tissue Salt*** Acts as a blood cleanser and good for skin, hair, and nails.

Athletes suffering from anemia, calcium deficiency, or any mineral deficiency or cramps can benefit from these salts. Please take the advice of a practitioner before taking tissue salts.

Gut Speaks

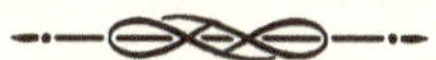

Your Gut answers your questions

Question-Should I count the calories I eat?

Answer- You don't need to count your calories. Here is a simple tip for you:

- Eat your food after 20 minutes when you get the hunger signal.
- Observe your plate. Ensure it has all the macro-nutrients (Fat, Proteins, Carbs) and the six tastes.
- Chew your food slowly; this gives enough time to signal the brain when one is full.
- Don't over-eat.

Question-How do I know I have eaten enough?

Answer- According to Ayurveda, when you get the full burp, it means you have eaten the right amount. Stop when you feel you are 75% full. If you feel sleepy after a heavy meal, you have eaten more.

Question-How to know what types of food suit me?

Answer- Please go through the dosha test as mentioned in the Ayurveda chapter and eat as per your constitution. Use the elimination technique. If some particular food causes gas, bloating, constipation, and other unpleasant feelings, it means that the food does not suit you. Refrain from having that kind of food or consult your dietician. Do not make drastic changes to your diet. Small changes over a few weeks will help give you the right signals.

Question-How do I know how much to drink in a day?

Answer- As per Ayurveda, we should be drinking water whenever we get thirsty; however that doesn't apply to athletes. Athletes' hydration requirements depend upon several factors like sweat rate, urine color, weather conditions. A simple rule is to check your urine color; if it's pale yellow, you need to hydrate more. Cucumber, Coconut water, watermelon are hydrating foods along with vital nutrients.

Question- How many hours before bedtime should one have dinner?

Answer- 3-4 hours before bedtime is ideal. Dinner should be light as compared to other meals. My digestive power is low post-sunset.

Question-Do you recommend a Vegan diet?

Answer- If you are allergic to milk and milk products, then yes. Moreover, if you have inflammatory conditions, then a vegan diet helps a lot. A vegan diet is very helpful for Arthritis patients.

Question-Do you recommend a Keto diet?

Answer- No, the keto diet strictly limits the intake of carbohydrates. By following the keto diet, some people experience headaches, nausea, vomiting, and other symptoms. This type of diet leads to vitamin/mineral deficiency. People are prone to kidney stones, fatty liver, hyperlipidemia. In the long run, it is challenging to follow this type of diet. Go for a wholesome diet that is sustainable.

Question-What is the optimum period for Intermittent Fasting?

Answer- You can do it anytime for a period of 14 to 18 hours. The optimum period for intermittent fasting is 16 hours.

Question-How to overcome constipation during Intermittent Fasting?

Answer- Drink plenty of water all day, especially during the fasting window. Have foods high in fiber and be physically active. Enema is a great way to clear the colon.

Question-What factors enable me to get adequate sleep at night?

Answer- Have dinner 3-4 hours before bedtime. Avoid all kinds of caffeinated beverages at night. Drink more fluids during the first half of the day compared to the second half. Foods containing tryptophan induce sleep. One can have a glass of warm milk with nutmeg and almonds. Chamomile tea stimulates sleep.

Question-What are the dietary changes for women undergoing menopause?

Answer- Increase your intake of calcium-rich foods, omega 3 fatty acids, essential amino acids, and anti-oxidants. Include fenugreek, flaxseeds, licorice in your diet. Avoid all kinds of sugary products and processed foods.

Question-How do I maintain healthy joints as I age?

Answer-Diet should be rich in Omega 3 fatty acids, vitamin D, calcium, vitamin K, and type II collagen (chicken broth). Any form of exercise is a must. Maintain a healthy weight.

Question-When do you recommend supplements?

Answer- Yes, when there are deficiencies. Vegetarians are more prone to vitamin B12 deficiency. If your blood test report shows a lack of any particular vitamin or mineral, do incorporate those supplements along with diet modifications. Cramping during runs indicates a deficiency of magnesium. Type II Collagen supplement is recommended for athletes after the age of 40.

Question-What are the signs of poor nutrition?

Answer- If one feels lethargic most of the time, the face looks dull, finds it difficult to do his/her regular activities, nails become brittle, rapid weight loss/gain. Bad cravings are also a sign of poor nutrition.

An athlete's poor nutrition signs are slow recovery, frequent cramps or injuries, morning fatigue, falling ill after a long workout. Lack of adequate sleep also causes all the above symptoms.

Homemade Energy Bar Recipes

Cut out hidden sugars, preservatives, and additives by making energy bars at home. Nutrient-dense bars are on-the-go snacks that will curb your hunger.

These bars can be refrigerated in an airtight container for up to a week or frozen in ziplock bags for up to a month. These bars are good pre-workout, during and post-workout, or on-the-go snacks. They're high in calories, so not advisable in larger quantities.

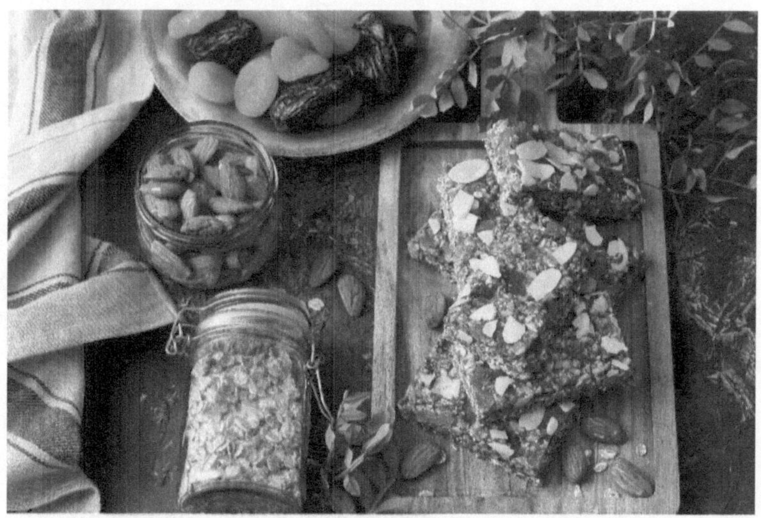

Picture 40: Homemade energy bars

Note: Some of the energy bar recipes have been sourced from the Times of India.[89]

Carrot Energy Squares

Prep: 10 mins; Cook: Nil (Makes 12 squares)

Ingredients

- ½ cup almonds
- ½ cup walnuts
- ½ cup raisins
- 1 cup carrots, grated
- 1 tbsp flax seeds, ground
- 2 dates, chopped
- 1 tbsp coconut oil
- ½ tsp lemon juice
- ¼ tsp pink salt
- grated dry coconut

Method

- Take almonds and walnuts in a food processor or blender and coarsely grind them.
- Add raisins, dates, and salt to the mix, and pulse again.
- Transfer the powder into a bowl and add grated carrots, flax seeds powder, coconut oil, and mix well.
- Spread the batter evenly on an aluminum foil and top it with grated dry coconut. Fold and refrigerate for half an hour.
- Remove and cut in squares. Keep refrigerated and use within a week.

Oats and Date Protein Bars

Prep: 10 mins; Cook: Nil (10-12 bars)

Ingredients

- ½ cup oats, powdered
- 1 cup of dates, pitted and chopped,
- ½ cup of almonds,
- 1 tbsp flax seeds,
- 1 tbsp sesame seeds,
- 1 tbsp coconut oil,
- 1 tbsp cocoa powder,
- 1 tsp cardamom powder,
- a pinch of sea salt

Method

- Crush almonds, flaxseeds and sesame seeds in a food processor till it forms a powder.
- Mix chopped dates, coconut oil, cocoa, cardamom powder, and oats.
- Pulse the mix till it forms a dough.
- Remove the dough, knead well and roll out on a greased surface into square shapes of 4-5 mm thickness.
- Cut into rectangles and store in an airtight container.

Milk and Cereal Bars

Prep: 10 mins; Cook: Nil; (Makes 5-6 bars)

Ingredients

- 1 cup Ragi flakes
- ½ cup packed oat flour
- ¼ tsp pink salt
- 2 tbsp milk powder
- 2 tbsp peanut butter
- 2 tbsp honey
- ¼ cup roasted almonds or coconut
- ¼ cup of Greek yogurt (optional)

Method

- Combine the ragi flakes, oat flour, and salt in a mixing bowl.
- In a separate bowl, combine the peanut butter, milk powder, and honey and mix it.
- Pour dry into wet ingredients and stir until even.
- Line a baking dish with a large piece of wax or parchment paper.
- Pour the batter into the dish. Using the second sheet of parchment, squish down as hard as you possibly can. Use a heavy object to press it down, if required.
- Sprinkle coconut or almond flakes on top and then put in the fridge or freezer to harden before cutting into bars.

Coconut & Millet Bars

Prep: 10 mins; Cook: 10 mins; (10 bars)

Ingredients

- 1 ½ cups puffed amaranth/rajgira
- ½ cup cocoa powder, a cup of honey
- 2 tbsp coconut oil

- 1 tsp vanilla extract
- 3 tbsp makhana, crushed
- ½ cup shredded coconut
- a pinch of pink salt

Method

- Dry roast coconut till it turns pink and keeps it aside.
- Dry roast amaranth for 5 minutes on slow flame and cool.
- Mix cocoa powder, oil, vanilla extract, and honey, and warm the mix till they are incorporated together.
- Add Amaranth and crushed makhana. Mix well.
- Line a baking pan with parchment paper. Grease the parchment paper with melted coconut oil.
- Place the chocolate-coated puffs into the lined baking dish and press down to create an even layer of puffs. Top with toasted coconut shreds.
- Place the pan in the freezer for about 20 minutes to allow the crisps to harden, then cut into desired shapes.

Apricot Bars

Prep: 10 mins; Cook: Nil; (Makes 5-6 bars)

Ingredients

- 1 cup Dried apricots
- 1 cup pitted dates
- 1 cup peanuts

Method

- Blend all ingredients in a processor.

- Spread it on butter paper in a pan.
- Refrigerate for an hour. Cut into pieces.

Amla bars

Prep: 10 mins; Cook: Nil; (Makes 5-6 bars)

Ingredients

- ½ cup dry amla candy
- 1 cup pitted dates
- 2 teaspoon peanut butter or almond butter

Method

- Blend all the ingredients in a blender.
- Spread it on a pan.
- Cut into desirable shapes after a few mins.

Date Rolls

Prep: 10 mins; Cook: Nil; (Makes 5-6 rolls)

Ingredients

- 1 cup pitted dates
- ½ cup almonds
- ¼ cup walnuts
- ¼ cup cashews

Method

- Blend the dates in a blender. Blend the nuts coarsely.
- Mix everything in a bowl.
- Apply ghee or butter to your hands.
- Roll it in well and refrigerate.

Biomarkers for Athletes

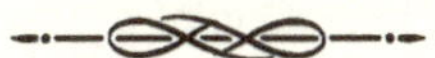

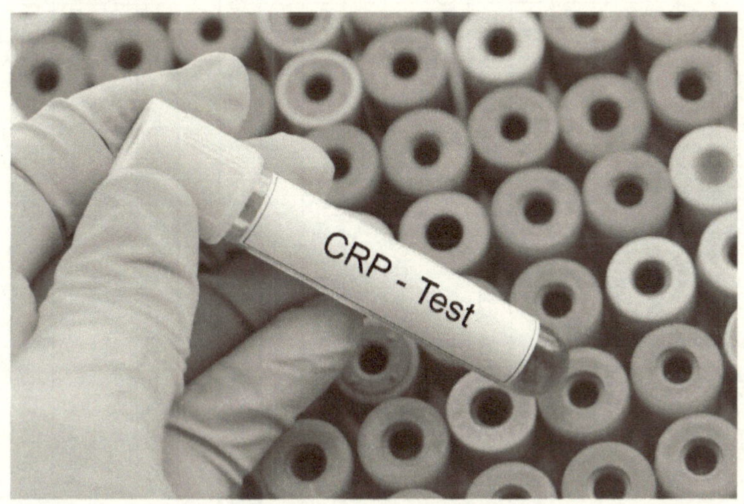

Picture 41: Biomarkers

Complete Blood Count	It is a group of tests to evaluate the cells that circulate in the blood, including red blood cells (RBCs), white blood cells (WBCs), and platelets (PLTs). The CBC can evaluate your overall health and detect various diseases and conditions, such as infections, anemia and leukemia.	
Biomarker	**Normal values for men**	**Normal values for women**
Hemoglobin (HGB)	13.8-17.2g/100ml	12.0-15.6g/100ml
Hematocrit	40-54%	38-46%
Red Blood Cells	4.4-5.8million/ml	3.9-5.2million/ml
White Blood Cells	3800-10.800ml	3800-10.800ml
Platelets	130.000-400.000/ml	130.000-400.000/ml
Lymphocytes	850-4100 cells/ml	850-4100 cells/ml
Neutrophils	1500-7800 cells/ml	1500-7800 cells/ml
Eosinophils	50-550 cells/ml	50-550 cells/ml
Basophils	0-200 cells/ml	0-200 cells/ml
Monocytes	200-1100 cells/ml	200-1100 cells/ml
MCH	27-32 picograms	27-32 picograms
MCHC	28-36g/100ml (RBC's only)	28-36g/100ml (RBC's only)
MCV	80-94 fl	80-94 fl
Muscle enzyme creatine kinase (CK)	38-174 units/L	90-140 units/L
myoglobin	10-95ng/mL	10-65ng/mL

Albumin	3.2-5.0gm/dL	3.2-5.0gm/dL
Fasting blood glucose	70-100mg/dL	70-100mg/dL
Random blood glucose	80-140mg/dL	80-140mg/dL
High-sensitivity C-reactive protein	less than 1.0 mg/L is ideal	Less than 1.0mg/L is ideal
BUN	6-23mg/dL	6-23mg/dL
Hemoglobin A1C (This is a measure of the average of the last 6-8 weeks of your blood sugar levels and can pick up metabolic syndrome and diabetes)	>5.5 % of total hemoglobin	>5.5 % of total hemoglobin
Uric acid	4.0-8.5mg/dL	2.5-7.5mg/dL
Homocysteine	less than 8.0 mmol/L is ideal	Less than 8.0mmol/L is ideal

Insulin Response Test	1 in 2 people have diabetes or metabolic syndrome (prediabetes), and 90% do not know it). The Insulin Response test is the best way to find out if you have a problem. Fasting and 1-hour and 2-hour glucose and insulin levels after a 75-gram glucose load.	
BioMarker	**Recommended Range**	
Fasting blood sugar	< 90 mg/dL	
One-hour and two-hour glucose	< 110 mg/dL	
Fasting insulin	Between 2 uIU/dL and 5, anything greater than 10 uIU/dL is significantly elevated.	
One-hour and two-hour insulin	Less than 25uIU/dL to 30uIU/dL. Anything higher than 30 uIU/dL indicates some degree of insulin resistance.	

Heart	This test measures the levels of cardiac biomarkers in your blood.
BioMarker	**Recommended Range**
ECG	Check with your physician.
TMT/Stress Test	Check with your physician.
2D Echo	Check with your physician.
Color Ultrasonic UCG	Check with your physician.
Calcium scan test	A score of zero is normal.

Thyroid Hormones	The thyroid gland releases triiodothyronine (T3) and thyroxine (T4) that play an important role in regulating your weight, energy levels, internal temperature, skin, hair, nail growth, etc.	
Biomarker	**Normal values for men**	**Normal values for women**
Free T3	80-190 ng/dL	80-190ng/dL
Free T4	4.5 – 12 ng/dL	4.5-12ng/dL
TSH	0.3 - 5.0mIU/L	0.3-5.0mIU/L
TPO Antibody	<15	<15

Cholesterol Panel	This test measures the amount of cholesterol and fats called triglycerides in the blood.	
Biomarker	**Normal values for men**	**Normal values for women**
Total cholesterol	> 180 mg/dL	>180mg/dL
LDL	>70 mg/dL	>70mg/dL
HDL cholesterol	<60 mg/dL	<60mg/dL
Triglycerides	>100 mg/dL	>100mg/dL
Triglyceride/HDL ratio	>4	>4
Total cholesterol/HDL ratio	>3	>3

NMR Lipid Profile	Particle size and number. Even if your cholesterol numbers are normal with or without medication, you may still be at significant risk if you have small cholesterol.
BioMarker	**Recommended Range**
Total LDL particles	< 1000 nmol/L
Total small LDL particles	< 600 nmol/L
LDL size	> 21 nm
HDL size	> 9 umol/L
VLDL	< 0.1 nmol/L

Vitamins and Minerals	These tests can detect gluten, mineral, iron, calcium, and other deficiencies, telling you which vitamins you lack.	
Biomarker	**Normal values for men**	**Normal values for women**
Vitamin D	20-50ng/mL	20-50ng/mL
Vitamin B12	200-900ng/mL	200-900ng/mL
Vitamin B6	5-50mcg/L	5-50mcg/L
Calcium	8.5-10.2mg/dL	8.5-10.2mg/dL
Iron	60-160mcg/dL	60-160mcg/dL
Sodium	135-148mEq/L	135-148mEq/L
Potassium	3.5-5.5mEq/L	3.5-5.5mEq/L
Magnesium	1.7 to 2.2 mg/dL	1.7 to 2.2 mg/dL
Chloride	96-112mEq/L	96-112mEq/L
Ferritin	10-350ng/mL	10-350ng/mL
Folate	4.0-20ng/mL	4.0-20ng/mL
Omega-6 to Omega-3 ratio	< 3:1.3	< 3:1.3

Hormone Panel	Hormones help control many of your body's major processes, including metabolism and reproduction. These tests are important in ensuring there are no hormone imbalances.	
BioMarker	**Normal values for men**	**Normal values for women**
Growth Hormone	<5ng/mL	<10ng/mL
Cortisol	10-20mcg/dL	10-20mcg/dL
Estrogen	10-60pg/mL	Depends upon age Women aged 20-29 have an average level of 149pg/mL (Aged 30-39)- 210pg/mL
Progesterone	NA	>75ng/mL
DHEA	7-31 nmol/L	
Testosterone	300-1200 ng/dL	8-60 ng/dL

Liver Function Tests	These tests identify the death of liver cells, most often caused by elevated insulin resistance because of a fatty liver	
Biomarker	**Normal values for men**	**Normal values for women**
Total protein	5.7-8.2gm/dL	5.7-8.2gm/dL
Alanine Aminotransferase (ALT)	29-33 IU/L	19-25 IU/L
Aspartate Aminotransferase (AST)	7-21 U/L	6-18 U/L
Gamma-glutamyl transpeptidase (GGT)	11-63 IU/L	8-35 IU/L

Kidney Function Tests [90]	Used to identify early damage to kidneys, which can occur from prediabetes, diabetes, and high blood pressure	
Biomarker	**Normal values for men**	**Normal values for women**
Urea Nitrogen	6-25mg/dL	6-20mg/dL
Creatinine	0.7-1.3 mg/dL	0.6-1.1 mg/dL
Urine microalbumin	Less than 30mcg/mg	Less than 30mcg/mg
Estimated GFR	100-130ml/min	90-120ml/min

Note: A reference range can vary between different laboratories. Please consult your family physician for the list of tests you need to do.

References

1. Going Paleo: What Prehistoric Man Actually Ate https://www.history.com/news/going-paleo-what-prehistoric-man-actually-ate

2. Neolithic Revolution https://www.history.com/topics/pre-history/neolithic-revolution

3. Breakfast, lunch and dinner: Have we always eaten them? https://www.bbc.com/news/magazine-20243692

4. Salt content of processed foods in India https://www.georgeinstitute.org/sites/default/files/salt-content-of-processed-foods-in-india-june-16.pdf

5. Defining the Human Microbiome https://www.ncbi.nlm.nih.gov/pmc/articles/PMC3426293/

6. Gut microbiota and Covid-19- possible link and implications https://www.ncbi.nlm.nih.gov/pmc/articles/PMC7217790/

7. Facing a new challenge: the adverse effects of antibiotics on gut microbiota and host immunity https://www.ncbi.nlm.nih.gov/pmc/articles/PMC6511407/

8. The Influence of Nonsteroidal Anti-Inflammatory Drugs on the Gut Microbiome https://www.ncbi.nlm.nih.gov/pmc/articles/PMC4754147/

9. The Western Diet–Microbiome-Host Interaction and Its Role in Metabolic Disease https://www.ncbi.nlm.nih.gov/pmc/articles/PMC5872783/

10. E. coli https://www.who.int/news-room/fact-sheets/detail/e-coli

11. Potential Causes and Consequences of Gastrointestinal Disorders during a SARS-CoV-2 Infection https://www.sciencedirect.com/science/article/pii/S2211124720308962

12. Stress Effects on the Body https://www.apa.org/helpcenter/stress/effects-gastrointestinal

13. Fermented Cereal-based Products: Nutritional Aspects, Possible Impact on Gut Microbiota and Health Implications https://www.researchgate.net/publication/341907432_Fermented_Cereal-based_Products_Nutritional_Aspects_Possible_Impact_on_Gut_Microbiota_and_Health_Implications

14. Antibacterial and Antifungal Activities of Spices https://www.ncbi.nlm.nih.gov/pmc/articles/PMC5486105/

15. Bacteriostatic effect of dill, fennel, caraway and cinnamon extracts against Helicobacter pylori https://www.researchgate.net/publication/232072333_Bacteriostatic_effect_of_dill_fennel_caraway_and_cinnamon_extracts_against_Helicobacter_pylori

16. Probiotics Prevent Dysbiosis and the Rise in Blood Pressure in Genetic Hypertension: Role of Short-Chain Fatty Acids https://pubmed.ncbi.nlm.nih.gov/31953983/

17. Prebiotics: Definition, Types, Sources, Mechanisms, and Clinical Applications https://www.ncbi.nlm.nih.gov/pmc/articles/PMC6463098/

18. Role of gut microbiota in cardiovascular diseases https://www.ncbi.nlm.nih.gov/pmc/articles/PMC7215967/

19. Postbiotics-parabiotics: the new horizons in microbial biotherapy and functional foods https://www.ncbi.nlm.nih.gov/pmc/articles/PMC7441679/

20. Building bridges between Ayurveda and Modern Science https://www.ncbi.nlm.nih.gov/pmc/articles/PMC2876924/

21. Bhagvad Gita Verse 17-07 http://www.bhagavad-gita.org/Gita/verse-17-07.html

22. Viruddha Ahara: A critical view https://www.ncbi.nlm.nih.gov/pmc/articles/PMC3665091/

23. Viruddhahara(Antagonistic food) https://www.nhp.gov.in/viruddhahara-antagonistic-food-_mtl

24. Role of Dinacharya Modalities in the Management of lifestyle disorders https://www.researchgate.net/publication/339643426_Role_of_Dinacharya_Modalities_in_the_Management_of_lifestyle_disorders

25. Oil pulling for maintaining oral hygiene – A review https://www.ncbi.nlm.nih.gov/pmc/articles/PMC5198813/

26. The Impact of Yoga Nidra and Seated Meditation on the Mental Health of College Professors https://www.ncbi.nlm.nih.gov/pmc/articles/PMC6134749/

27. Five step protocol for a healthy living https://youtu.be/M58SRlk2IHc

28. Health Hazards Of Sulphur In Sugar https://ehealth.eletsonline.com/2014/01/health-hazards-of-sulphur-in-sugar/

29. A review of permissible limits of drinking water https://www.ncbi.nlm.nih.gov/pmc/articles/PMC3482709/

30. Over 100,000 infants in India did not survive a month due to severe air pollution in 2019: Report https://www.hindustantimes.com/india-news/over-100-000-infants-in-india-did-not-survive-a-month-due-to-severe-air-pollution-in-2019-report/story-EaUP0546eW2ghlWrfominO.html

31. Arsenic, Lead Found in Popular Protein Supplements https://www.consumerreports.org/dietary-supplements/heavy-metals-in-protein-supplements/

32. Toxicity, mechanism and health effects of some heavy metals https://www.ncbi.nlm.nih.gov/pmc/articles/PMC4427717/

33. Bisphenol A (BPA) https://www.niehs.nih.gov/health/topics/agents/sya-bpa/index.cfm

34. A review of the occurrence of pharmaceuticals and personal care products in Indian water bodies https://www.researchgate.net/publication/311425932_A_review_of_the_occurrence_of_pharmaceuticals_and_personal_care_products_in_Indian_water_bodies

35. Health effects of environmental pollution in population living near industrial complex areas in Korea https://www.ncbi.nlm.nih.gov/pmc/articles/PMC5903037/

36. The Effect of Nasal Breathing Versus Oral and Oronasal Breathing During Exercise: A Review https://www.researchgate.net/publication/338558548_The_Effect_of_Nasal_Breathing_Versus_Oral_and_Oronasal_Breathing_During_Exercise_A_Review

37. Importance of Nasya in Today's Era: A Practical Approach http://www.ccras.nic.in/node/1200

38. Pratimarsha Nasya http://www.ccras.nic.in/node/1060

39. Physiology, Acid Base Balance https://www.ncbi.nlm.nih.gov/books/NBK507807/

40. "Cleanse" detoxification diet program in Appalachia: Participant characteristics and perceived health effects https://pubmed.ncbi.nlm.nih.gov/31536033/

41. Principles of Fasting in Ayurveda https://www.researchgate.net/publication/313250061_Principles_of_Fasting_in_Ayurveda

42. Research on intermittent fasting shows health benefits https://www.nia.nih.gov/news/research-intermittent-fasting-shows-health-benefits

43. What happens if you fast for a day? https://www.medicalnewstoday.com/articles/322065

44. Alternate-day fasting in nonobese subjects: effects on body weight, body composition, and energy metabolism https://academic.oup.com/ajcn/article/81/1/69/4607679

45. A Time to Eat and a Time to Exercise https://journals.lww.com/acsm-essr/fulltext/2020/01000/a_time_to_eat_and_a_time_to_exercise.3.aspx

46. Effects of a 3-day fast on regional lipid and glucose metabolism in human skeletal muscle and adipose tissue https://www.researchgate.net/publication/6055419_Effects_of_a_3-day_fast_on_regional_lipid_and_glucose_metabolism_in_human_skeletal_muscle_and_adipose_tissue

47. Everything You Want to Know About Dry Fasting https://www.healthline.com/health/food-nutrition/dry-fasting

48. A glycaemic index compendium of non-western foods https://pubmed.ncbi.nlm.nih.gov/33414403/

49. Nutrition and Supplement Update for the Endurance Athlete: Review and Recommendations https://www.ncbi.nlm.nih.gov/pmc/articles/PMC6628334/

50. How to use Amino Acids https://bengreenfieldfitness.com/article/supplements-articles/how-to-use-amino-acids/

51. Product Development, Biochemical and Organoleptic Analysis of a Sports Drink https://www.iosrjournals.org/iosr-jspe/papers/vol1-issue4/A0140105.pdf

52. Does coffee ACTUALLY dehydrate you and harm your performance? https://www.precisionhydration.com/performance-advice/hydration/does-coffee-dehydrate-you/

53. Dehydration and endurance performance in competitive athletes https://www.researchgate.net/publication/264720964_Dehydration_and_endurance_performance_in_competitive_athletes

54. Muscle Cramping During Exercise: Causes, Solutions, and Questions Remaining https://link.springer.com/article/10.1007/s40279-019-01162-1

55. Glutamine as an Anti-Fatigue Amino Acid in Sports Nutrition https://www.ncbi.nlm.nih.gov/pmc/articles/PMC6520936/

56. Effects of Arginine Supplementation on Athletic Performance Based on Energy Metabolism: A Systematic Review and Meta-Analysis https://www.ncbi.nlm.nih.gov/pmc/articles/PMC7282262/

57. Glutathione supplementation suppresses muscle fatigue induced by prolonged exercise via improved aerobic metabolism https://www.ncbi.nlm.nih.gov/pmc/articles/PMC4328900/

58. 24-Week study on the use of collagen hydrolysate as a dietary supplement in athletes with activity-related joint pain https://pubmed.ncbi.nlm.nih.gov/18416885/

59. Effects of Ashwagandha (Withania somnifera) on VO2max: A Systematic Review and Meta-Analysis https://www.researchgate.net/publication/340838628_Effects_of_Ashwagandha_Withania_somnifera_on_VO2max_A_Systematic_Review_and_Meta-Analysis

60. Characterisation of polyphenols in Terminalia arjuna bark extract https://www.ijpsonline.com/articles/characterisation-of-polyphenols-in-terminalia-arjuna-bark-extract.html

61. Triphala: current applications and new perspectives on the treatment of functional gastrointestinal disorders https://cmjournal.biomedcentral.com/articles/10.1186/s13020-018-0197-6

62. Moringa oleifera: a health food for animal and human consumption https://www.researchgate.net/publication/338914349_Moringa_oleifera_a_health_food_for_animal_and_human_consumption

63. Curcumin: An age-old anti-inflammatory and anti-neoplastic agent https://www.sciencedirect.com/science/article/pii/S22254110016302528

64. Asparagus racemosus (Shatavari): A Versatile Female Tonic https://www.researchgate.net/publication/258448671_Asparagus_racemosus_Shatavari_A_Versatile_Female_Tonic

65. Biomarkers in Sports and Exercise: Tracking Health, Performance, and Recovery in Athletes https://www.ncbi.nlm.nih.gov/pmc/articles/PMC5640004/

66. 5 Foods That Can Cause Inflammation https://health.clevelandclinic.org/5-foods-that-can-cause-inflammation/

67. Design of an anti-inflammatory diet (ITIS diet) for patients with rheumatoid arthritis https://www.ncbi.nlm.nih.gov/pmc/articles/PMC6997513/

68. Potential role of bromelain in clinical and therapeutic applications https://www.ncbi.nlm.nih.gov/pmc/articles/PMC4998156/

69. Turmeric Potential Health Benefits https://journals.lww.com/nutritiontodayonline/fulltext/2020/01000/turmeric__potential_health_benefits.9.aspx

70. The Potential Benefits of Red Beetroot Supplementation in Health and Disease https://www.researchgate.net/publication/275032768_The_Potential_Benefits_of_Red_Beetroot_Supplementation_in_Health_and_Disease

71. Beneficial effects of walnut consumption on human health https://journals.lww.com/co-clinicalnutrition/

fulltext/2018/11000/beneficial_effects_of_walnut_
consumption_on_human.15.aspx

72. Leafy greens linked with slower age-related cognitive decline
    https://www.nia.nih.gov/news/leafy-greens-linked-slower-age-
    related-cognitive-decline

73. Broccoli and Cruciferous Vegetables: Reduce Overall Cancer
    Risk   https://www.aicr.org/cancer-prevention/food-facts/
    broccoli-cruciferous-vegetables/

74. What's New and Beneficial About Flaxseeds http://www.
    whfoods.com/genpage.php?tname=foodspice&dbid=81

75. Ubiquinol supplementation enhances peak power production in
    trained athletes: a double-blind, placebo controlled study https://
    jissn.biomedcentral.com/articles/10.1186/1550-2783-10-24

76. Effects of acute and 14-day coenzyme Q10 supplementation on
    exercise performance in both trained and untrained individuals
    https://www.ncbi.nlm.nih.gov/pmc/articles/PMC2315638/

77. Boswellia   Serrata,   A   Potential   Antiinflammatory
    Agent: An   Overview   https://www.researchgate.net/
    publication/223137254_Boswellia_Serrata_A_Potential_
    Antiinflammatory_Agent_An_Overview

78. Iron leaf shakti https://weisheithome.com/product/lucky-
    shakti-leaf/

79. Dietary Guidelines for Indiana https://www.nin.res.in/
    downloads/DietaryGuidelinesforNINwebsite.pdf

80. What is the Endocrine System? https://www.epa.gov/
    endocrine-disruption/what-endocrine-system

81. Hypothyroidism and obesity: An intriguing link https://www.
    ncbi.nlm.nih.gov/pmc/articles/PMC4911848/

82. The role of micronutrients in thyroid dysfunction https://
    www.ncbi.nlm.nih.gov/pmc/articles/PMC7282437/

83. GREEN COFFEE IN PHARMACEUTICAL INDUSTRY: A BOON TO MANKIND http://ijiset.com/vol7/v7s8/IJISET_V7_I8_15.pdf

84. The Role of Environmental Pollution in Endocrine Diseases https://link.springer.com/referenceworkentry/10.1007%2F978-3-319-66362-3_16-1

85. HORMONAL CHANGES AT REST IN OVERTRAINED ENDURANCE ATHLETES https://www.ncbi.nlm.nih.gov/pmc/articles/PMC7098450/

86. Effects of Alcohol on the Endocrine System https://www.ncbi.nlm.nih.gov/pmc/articles/PMC3767933/

87. Alcohol: Impact on Sports Performance and Recovery in Male Athleteshttps://www.researchgate.net/publication/261761789_Alcohol_Impact_on_Sports_Performance_and_Recovery_in_Male_Athletes

88. Migraine relief: Try these roll-ons, patches & more https://timesofindia.indiatimes.com/most-searched-products/health-and-fitness/health-care/migraine-relief-try-these-oils-roll-ons-more-to-get-relief-in-migraine-pain/articleshow/72110924.cms

89. Cell Salt Therapy https://www.encyclopedia.com/medicine/encyclopedias-almanacs-transcripts-and-maps/cell-salt-therapy

90. Try these 5 energy bar recipes for an instant boost! https://timesofindia.indiatimes.com/life-style/food-news/feeling-tired-all-the-time-try-these-5-energy-bar-recipes-for-an-instant-boost/photostory/76722975.cms?picid=76723009

91. Renal Function Tests https://www.ncbi.nlm.nih.gov/books/NBK507821/